ATTITUDES IN PSYCHIATRIC NURSING CARE

Attitudes in Psychiatric Nursing Care

MADELINE OLGA WEISS, R.N., B.Sc., M.Litt.

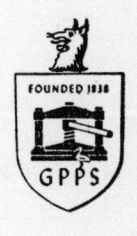

G. P. PUTNAM'S SONS   New York

COPYRIGHT, 1954, BY G. P. PUTNAM'S SONS

All rights reserved. This book, or parts thereof, must not be reproduced in any form without permission. Published simultaneously in the Dominion of Canada by McAinsh & Co., Limited, Toronto.

Third Printing

MANUFACTURED IN THE UNITED STATES OF AMERICA

VAN REES PRESS • NEW YORK

Preface

THE NURSING PROFESSION recognizes more and more the need to approach patients as persons whose problems are more than those evidenced by the symptoms of the immediate physical illness. It is my hope that this book will help all who work with patients to understand why sick persons act the way they do, and how the attitudes of the personnel may affect recovery.

The book is an attempt to put into writing in elaborated and expanded form some of the ideas on which the medical and nursing staffs at the Menninger Sanitarium and Clinic worked for many hours and months. I was a member of the nursing staff at that time, when attitudes as a part of psychiatric treatment were neither generally accepted nor generally used elsewhere. Out of the conferences and discussions, the booklet *Guide to Physician's Orders* evolved. Permission to use the *Guide* is gratefully acknowledged.

My deepest thanks are extended to Dr. Karl and Dr. William Menninger, tireless teachers and good friends, whose encouragement and guidance have motivated my efforts in preparing this work. Thanks, too, are due the editors of the *American Journal of Nursing* for their encouragement and support, and to those nurses and friends who have read the manuscript in part and in whole, and who gave such constructive criticism.

Every teaching project has goals; the following are the objectives of this treatise on attitudes in psychiatric nursing care:

Central Objective:

To stimulate interest in and to acquire knowledge of attitudes as therapy in nursing care

Contributory Objectives:

To gain knowledge of what is meant by attitudes
To gain awareness of how we acquire attitudes
To gain ability in utilizing attitudes
To gain skill in recognizing all the needs of sick persons in the home, the community, and the hospital
To gain in professional growth through the application of sound mental-hygiene principles in daily living
To give better nursing care to all sick persons

Although each of us is an individual, we live as members of a group, and how we get along in that group determines our happiness and success. We hear a great deal these days of how to get along with others and be successful in our daily lives. Perhaps it would be wise to decide just what success is and how we measure it. Success means many things to many people, but essentially it means enjoying one's life and, at the same time, being accepted by the group with whom we have the closest contact. How can we enjoy life when we must consider the feelings of all these other persons, when such consideration means curbing some of our own strongest desires and wants? We cultivate attitudes, which means, according to our standard English dictionaries, a position or stand, assumed or studied, to serve a purpose. This position, stand, or attitude shifts with each contact we make, and, since in modern life we encounter many varied people and situations, we must keep a supply or stock of attitudes on hand for constant use. We are not conscious of this supply, but we can call certain attitudes into consciousness without much effort once we have an idea of how they will affect specific persons and situations. Essentially, attitudes are tools for building our lives.

We are familiar with the words and, indeed, have probably said of another, "It wasn't what he said, but the way he said

PREFACE

it, that upset me." Or we have had to explain that something we said or did was misinterpreted because of the attitude we seemed to have taken. We shall review attitudes in this book and attempt to strengthen the reader's understanding of those basic ones we all have toward people and situations in our present-day society. The most fundamental of these is related to acceptance; by our acceptance or nonacceptance of the world around us, we build our lives. We accept those people we love and those situations which are pleasant. We may also accept people and situations we know well, even if no great pleasure is associated with them. We may get annoyed or irritated with them at times, but, because they are familiar, we accept them, for it is easier to accept the known than to face the unknown. People or situations which are a part of a life pattern necessary to our existence are accepted even when they are unpleasant, sometimes because we know no alternative. Acceptance, then, is the basic attitude in our living, and once we have accepted ourselves and can be accepting of others, we can utilize other attitudes. Accepting ourselves and our relation to others indicates that we have reached a state of maturity in which we are able to meet people or situations we don't like, without suffering a sense of guilt requiring punishment. We make certain adjustments in our attitudes and reactions so that such meetings can be pleasant and productive.

Although the nurse frequently encounters situations which are not to her liking, there are attitudes which she can use that will make her more comfortable in her work and, at the same time, help her provide the very best of patient care. There are numerous psychiatric-nursing textbooks which describe disease conditions, the physical care of patients with these conditions, and the routines of psychiatric-hospital nursing. This book will discuss only attitudes which will help us to understand a bit better our fellow beings, regardless of the official diagnosis given them. It is believed these attitudes will prove useful in any nursing situation, whether in a psychiatric hospital or in a general hospital.

M. O. W.

Foreword

THERE WAS A TIME in the history of nursing when to fetch and carry was a nurse's chief function. Her feet were her most important qualification. As nursing techniques developed, especially in surgery, the nurse's hands became more important. Then came the emphasis upon knowledge, and nurses were taught anatomy and physiology and pharmacology (and *sometimes* even had one lecture on psychology!). The nurse's brain became the most important organ in her qualifications.

In the modern psychiatric hospital, more important than her feet, or her hands, or her brain, are the manifestations of the nurse's heart. What she *is* will do more for the healing of the patients in her charge than what she does or what she knows. If she has the maturity and the deep inner wisdom to be able to love even the people she doesn't like, she will be a good psychiatric nurse and she will help frightened, desperate, hopeless patients to get well.

The question arises as to whether the brain can influence the heart, and the heart influence the brain, in the direction of hands and feet and voice. Can we, in other words, teach a nurse (and teach ourselves if we are doctors) to be selective in the expression of our feelings and attitudes in a way that fits the patient's specific needs? Sympathy is a *sine qua non* of nursing, but the *expression* of sympathy can be a restoring balm *or* an aggravating encouragement of unhealthy tendencies. Cheerful enthusiasm may be inspiring or maddening. Some individuals have intuitive gifts of knowing when to contain themselves and when to express an attitude and, if the latter, which attitude. For toward every act of a fellow man, there are always in each of us several attitudes, sometimes conflictual. But not everyone is intuitively able to make the wisest choice, especially in dealing with the mentally sick, where it is so important.

Miss Weiss has had years of experience and has given many hours of thought to this problem. I remember her as an earnest, cooperative staff member in the Menninger Psychiatric Hospital when my brother Will was endeavoring to discover a way to improve the emotional disciplining of the staff and the teaching of helpful attitudes to new nurses and doctors. I am glad she has written out and elaborated these ideas. No one knows better than she the objections, the difficulties, the deficiencies in her text. But no young nurse who studies her book could be other than helped to be more helpful to her patients. It is in this way that the brain can help the heart to help the mind.

Karl A. Menninger, M.D.

Contents

	PAGE
Preface	v
Foreword	ix

CHAPTER

1 What Are Attitudes?   3
    Active Friendliness   3
    Indulgence or Permissiveness   4
    Passive Friendliness   5
    Watchfulness   6
    Matter-of-factness   7
    Firmness   7

2 Attitudes as Therapy   10
    Staff Attitudes   10
    Patients' Attitudes   11
    Admission Procedure   11
    Nurse-Patient Relationship   13

3 Some Safety Factors in Mental Hospitals   18
    Use of Equipment   19
    Restraints   23

4 The Art of Answering Questions   28
    What Patients' Questions Mean   29
    Answering Questions by Asking a Question   31
    Direct Answers   32
    Referral to Other Sources   33
    Offering Help in Getting Answers   34

CHAPTER		PAGE
5	**General Attitudes Used**	36
	Security and Protection	37
	Helpfulness	40
	Permissiveness	41
	Matter-of-factness	43
	Kind Firmness	44
	Is an Assumed Attitude Honest?	45
6	**Specific Attitudes**	48
	The Schizophrenic Patient	48
	The Depressed Patient	54
	Anxiety and Fear	60
	The Psychoneurotic Patient	61
	The Feeble-minded Patient	64
	Organic Brain Damage	67
	Behavior Problems	68
7	**Psychotic Children**	78
	Abnormal Behavior	78
	Nursing Techniques	80
	Emotional Entanglements	93
8	**Love, the Basis of Attitude Therapy**	96
	Rejection	97
	The Hospital Group	98
9	**The Nurse as an Individual**	101
	Responsibility to One's Self	102
	Responsibility to Society	104
Index		109

Contents

	PAGE
Preface	v
Foreword	ix

CHAPTER

1 What Are Attitudes?   3
    Active Friendliness   3
    Indulgence or Permissiveness   4
    Passive Friendliness   5
    Watchfulness   6
    Matter-of-factness   7
    Firmness   7

2 Attitudes as Therapy   10
    Staff Attitudes   10
    Patients' Attitudes   11
    Admission Procedure   11
    Nurse-Patient Relationship   13

3 Some Safety Factors in Mental Hospitals   18
    Use of Equipment   19
    Restraints   23

4 The Art of Answering Questions   28
    What Patients' Questions Mean   29
    Answering Questions by Asking a Question   31
    Direct Answers   32
    Referral to Other Sources   33
    Offering Help in Getting Answers   34

CHAPTER		PAGE
5	**General Attitudes Used**	36
	Security and Protection	37
	Helpfulness	40
	Permissiveness	41
	Matter-of-factness	43
	Kind Firmness	44
	Is an Assumed Attitude Honest?	45
6	**Specific Attitudes**	48
	The Schizophrenic Patient	48
	The Depressed Patient	54
	Anxiety and Fear	60
	The Psychoneurotic Patient	61
	The Feeble-minded Patient	64
	Organic Brain Damage	67
	Behavior Problems	68
7	**Psychotic Children**	78
	Abnormal Behavior	78
	Nursing Techniques	80
	Emotional Entanglements	93
8	**Love, the Basis of Attitude Therapy**	96
	Rejection	97
	The Hospital Group	98
9	**The Nurse as an Individual**	101
	Responsibility to One's Self	102
	Responsibility to Society	104

Index   109

ATTITUDES IN PSYCHIATRIC NURSING CARE

CHAPTER 1

What Are Attitudes?

NURSING CARE INVOLVES the use of attitudes in giving patients the greatest opportunity to regain their health and to learn good health habits. Just as we apply dressings and give specific medications, we may also use certain attitudes to aid patients.

The attitudes described here are used by all of us throughout the day—with one another, with the patients, with visitors, with every person we contact. Even a smile is an expression of an attitude. Because of their seeming simplicity, we may forget how important attitudes are in our work, especially with mentally ill patients. In the sections that follow, attitudes essential to good nursing care are named, and characterized in some detail.

Active Friendliness

Active friendliness means an attitude of interest in the immediate well-being of the patient, despite the attitude the patient himself may be presenting. It implies being ready and able to discuss sincerely his activities in the hospital and at home, giving attention to his needs without waiting for an expression of them. For example, the nurse may suggest, "It's a lovely day—just right for a walk outdoors," or "Would you like a glass of fruit juice?" or "I just saw the menu for lunch; it looks good."

The important basic principle in active friendliness is giving attention *before* the patient requests it, and means (as with all attitudes) that the hour of the day or night has nothing to do with its use as therapy. Common sense and a genuine interest in the patient as a person guide the nurse in its use.

Although the nurse should be ready always to show friendly interest, the reality of necessary hospital routine must not be neglected, but it should never be used as an excuse to sever contact with the patient; that is, the nurse does not rush through the personal-hygiene routine, sign supply forms, give medications, and then drop her busy air and become a friendly person. Routines can be carried out with somewhat less formality and rigidity than is often common in the hospital. If a patient does not care to brush his teeth at a specified time, there is no real reason for insisting that he do so, and the nurse need not act like a punishing mother because her routine did not function smoothly. For some patients, active friendliness is not effective. We shall discuss this later in the explanation of other attitudes.

Summed up, active friendliness means a consistent genuine interest in the patient and his activities twenty-four hours a day. It means seeking out the patient, commending him for his achievements, however minor, and giving him extra attention and companionship.

Indulgence or Permissiveness

Some patients are so frightened of reality, even the reality of a protective place like the psychiatric hospital, that it is necessary for us to accept behavior normally unacceptable in most groups. This is permissiveness or indulgence. It means that the nurse accepts, without punishing, minor infractions of the ward rules; she may even instigate such infractions, for example, by allowing the patient to sit by her desk and read after "lights out" at night. She does this not on the basis of her own like or dislike of a patient but on the order or suggestion of the physician or supervisor, because she is aware of the patient's need for indulgence, and so that he may learn that people accept him and like him. It is basically a form of reassurance to the patient, an encouragement to be an individual and to learn to trust the hospital personnel. This attitude may be changed later, as may all attitudes, when the patient has improved enough to meet reality without fear. Patients often need to be protected from hostility expressed by other patients or by themselves; that is, their occasional expressions of hostility should be met without comment or punishment. This permissiveness supports and aids them to recognize that expressions of aggression (and they are often mild) will not always alienate people or result in some fearful calamity. With recognition of this, they often begin to feel more secure and have less need for the frequent use of hostile expressions and attitudes to test those around them.

Passive Friendliness

Passive friendliness implies an attitude of interest in the patient's welfare, but one which does not seek him out to reassure him of that friendliness. Rather, the nurse is friendly when the patient approaches her at any time, shows an interest, but allows, indeed encourages, the patient to make the initial overtures. This is familiar to all of us, since it is simply what we do with many of the people we meet in our daily lives. We like them and are pleased when they see us and stop for a chat, but we do not seek them out, call to invite them to join us at a movie, or make any active overtures. Such friendliness is implied but is not pushed.

Patients for whom this attitude is employed are often people who are frightened by active friendly attentions, who recognize some of their own emotional reactions, and who will seek the friendship, attention, or companionship of the nurse when they need it but will be dismayed or angered (which means they have been frightened) if the nurse initiates the attention. These persons often feel that as long as the nurse is silent they are improving. They will usually carry out the daily routines of the hospital and their own activities without much thought or expectation of active friendliness from the nursing staff. Passivity is a difficult thing for nurses to manage at times—nurses seem to have bred into them a great need for action—and passive friendliness is difficult to maintain. It is important to remember that such an attitude must be kept below the point of hostilely ignoring all the activity of the patients for whom this attitude is suggested.

Watchfulness

Watchfulness is the first rule of all psychiatric hospitals, but there will be certain patients for whom this will be ordered especially. It may be called suicidal precautions, constant observation, twenty-four-hour companionship, or some other name, but it means constant vigilance. Patients for whom watchfulness is ordered are considered serious elopement or suicidal risks. Here the responsibility is in the hands of the personnel throughout the hospital, and the nurse on the ward must know at all times where such patients are and what they are doing. The important point in assuming an attitude of watchfulness is to be as matter-of-fact and as secure about it as possible. If the nurse cannot feel secure in watching patients, her insecurity is pretty sure to be picked up by the patient, who is sensitive to attitudes even though he may not understand their therapeutic use. Patients for whom this attitude is ordered usually feel more secure when they know they are being watched, even though they may express hostility to the personnel for being there so constantly, and even though they may try every trick and device they can think of to evade the observation of the hospital staff. This can get to be a game of the patient's attempting to outwit the nurse, and the nurse must be constantly alert to prevent the patient's winning such a game, where the stake may be his life. The attitude implies, too, more than watching the patient alone; the personnel must be aware of the many tools of daily hospital life which can prove dangerous to the life of such persons, and frequent inspection should be made of the patient's belongings, as well as the hospital ward itself, for any article secreted to aid the patient to escape, harm others, or commit suicide.

Matter-of-factness

Matter-of-factness is a simple attitude, yet it is one which nurses seem to find difficult to use as much as they could. From a negative point of view, it means not getting defensive about the hospital routines, the orders, or the treatment the nurse must carry out. More positively, it means an acceptance of one's self and one's role by carrying out the necessary duties pleasantly and calmly. Patients for whom this attitude is necessary are often nagging and complaintive and may make frequent bids for sympathy, whether because of physical pain or because of some (to them) annoying hospital routine. The nurse should ignore all such bids, go on about her routines, and be friendly toward the patient. She should avoid falling into the trap of arguing or defending the hospital, the diet kitchen, or the doctor's orders. "This is the way it is, so we accept it" should be implied by her calm manner in carrying out the daily routines.

Firmness

Firmness is another attitude difficult for nurses to assume, since they frequently interpret it to mean sternness or cruelty to the patient. Some patients, usually the self-punitive, suicidal persons, cannot accept overt friendliness. They feel unworthy, guilty, or fearful, and active or even passive friendliness adds to, rather than lessens, the burden of their guilt. The attitude of firmness implies a near sternness in the care of such patients, but the nurse must be careful not to use this attitude to express some of her own hostility. Firmness is a tool for the care of the patient only—not a release for the nurse's own tensions.

Requests for punishment, such as "Let me go out and freeze," "Let me starve," "The food is too good to be served to me," and the countless depressed and self-punitive remarks such patients make, should be ignored when possible, or attention should be diverted from them. Tasks given to these patients are good methods of diversion and may be simple but monotonous duties such as drawing lines on charts for the nursing staff, folding dressings, weeding the walks, or rolling a tennis court, depending on the patient's physical condition and ability, the doctor's orders, the facilities available, and the nurse's ingenuity. Such patients also may have outbursts of aggression which should be restricted firmly. The patient should be told that his hostile speeches in the lounge or his physical attacks on others (if he makes them) are not acceptable, and there must be enough personnel on hand to meet such hostility promptly, firmly, and kindly, by diversion if possible. If actual physical force is needed, it should be well planned, smoothly run, and used with a minimum of comment; it must be firm and prompt. Once over, the incident should be forgotten, nor should it be referred to by the nurse at any future time. If the patient refers to the incident later, the nurse should change the subject tactfully or reassure the patient by letting him know in some way that the outburst was a part of his illness.

Some of these attitudes all of us assume in our daily lives, either in the hospital or at home. There are other gradations which may be altered to fit the individual and the situation in which they are needed. Mainly, it is important to recognize that the needs of the basic personality of the patient are what we must meet, despite the diagnosis, whether in or out of the hospital. The schizophrenic is frightened, afraid of reality, afraid of being disliked, afraid of being laughed at. Hence, to combat that fear we must be actively friendly. If he is so frightened that friendliness makes him withdraw further, we must continue being friendly, but rather watchfully so, letting our interest in him be so close to the surface that he may be sure of it even at his most withdrawn moments, but not pressing attention upon him if we see the signs of fright and withdrawal increasing. The depressed patient is fearful too, but he has converted his fright and anger into the desire to be punished. This should be met with firmness and a rigid control of the situation in order to show him that we will not allow him to injure himself, or to get pleasure from his discomfort.

SUGGESTED REFERENCES

Guide to the Order Sheet (mimeographed pamphlet), The Menninger Foundation, Topeka, Kans., 1946, pp. 8–32.

Hinsie, Leland, *The Person in the Body*, W. W. Norton & Company, New York, 1945.

Menninger, William C., *Fundamentals of Psychiatry*, Capper Printing Co., Topeka, Kans., 1943.

Webster's Collegiate Dictionary, 5th ed., G. & C. Merriam Company, Springfield, Mass., 1944.

Weiss, M. Olga, "Attempted Suicide—Then What?" *American Journal of Nursing*, 49:290, 1949.

CHAPTER 2

Attitudes as Therapy

WE HAVE DISCUSSED in the preceding chapter what some of the attitudes imply and how they may be utilized in the care of patients. This chapter will show more explicitly how attitudes are used by all of us, and how knowledge and awareness of them can be useful in treating patients.

Staff Attitudes

The graduate nurse in a psychiatric hospital is there, we assume, because psychiatric nursing appeals to her, and she has a working knowledge of the mental illnesses and how to nurse them. The student nurse is there to gain a working knowledge of mental illness. While initially she may have some fear and even disgust, her quest of knowledge has led her into this situation. Her attitude is one of seeking knowledge, plus the desire to be of service to the patients. Security and liking for the field are necessary to overcome fear and disgust, and security will come with familiarity and knowledge. Other personnel—the ward aides, orderlies, maids, and janitors—are necessary to the maintenance of complete service to the sick. They should have some teaching as to why patients are in mental hospitals and why they behave as they do. Those who work in hospitals are employed to give service to the sick, and good service demands an interest in and a knowledge of the job to be done. The student or graduate nurse should act as an interpreter to such personnel, as well as to families and other visitors. If, after the first few weeks of work, anyone employed in a mental hospital still is unhappy or frightened in his work, it is best to find employment elsewhere or to seek help from the personnel director, supervisor, or physician.

Patients' Attitudes

The patient enters the psychiatric hospital with all sorts of fears and misinformation superimposed upon an illness which carries its own fears and dreads. Many patients have never been in a hospital and haven't the slightest idea of what to expect. Those who have been in general hospitals have learned a routine of physical care and attention which is far different from the type of attention and care given in a psychiatric unit. As we can expect, then, the patient enters the psychiatric hospital with fear, ignorance of treatment methods, and often hostility toward his family and the hospital personnel. These fears must be allayed at once, and the nurse's attitude when she first meets the patient is of paramount importance.

Admission Procedure

The first thing that happens to patients in mental hospitals is the admission routine. It varies from hospital to hospital, but essentially it is the same: that is, the person is recognized, or recognizes himself, as being ill and in need of treatment in a hospital. All hospitals have routines set up to simplify care of groups of sick people, maintain safety within the group, and aid in the recovery and resocialization of sick persons. The initial contact with hospital personnel can establish a good or poor basis for accepting and responding to this care. The nurse should introduce herself, then introduce the patient to other ward personnel as well as to any patients who may be there. This is simple courtesy and should be expected of any hostess who has a guest in her charge for any length of time. It is a normal routine of human life, one that the patient will expect, either consciously or unconsciously.

Since this situation usually will be a new one to the patient, a good bit of explanation will be needed. Some hospitals use a printed booklet to explain the major portion of the routines and procedures; many do not. In either case, a personal explanation from the admitting nurse is advisable and courteous. The patient's fears may or may not be expressed, but the nurse should explain matter-of-factly and pleasantly that this is where the patient will be living for a while. If the building is locked, she should tell him this and explain the system for the patients' leaving a locked building. For example, "After we get to know you and you get to know us, you may be given permission to leave the building. For a while, you may be accompanied—it is easy to get lost in a new place, and someone from the staff will escort you to the various buildings and wards where you may have to go. Later on, you may be permitted to go out alone." (Here an explanation of that hospital's privilege or responsibility system may be made.) "You may be moved to another building where the doors remain unlocked, and, eventually, you may even attend the day hospital, or live in town and come to the outpatient clinic. That will be decided after you have been studied and we all know what is the best treatment for you."

The patient now knows immediately some of the more frightening details of the psychiatric hospital. He may ask about the "bad" patients, the excited patients, etc., expecting to see padded cells, dungeons, and goodness only knows what other horrors. This is normal, and is the impression of mental hospitals held by many lay persons and even by professional persons unfamiliar with psychiatry. Such fears should not be laughed at, for ridicule at this time, or any time, only creates feelings of hostility and may hinder treatment. If necessary, the nurse may talk about "crazy" people: she may explain that we don't think of people as being crazy but, rather, that they are ill, and that the nurses are there to help them get well, using all the latest knowledge and equipment. After this reassurance, she should make an explanation of the various hospital routines, showing the patient, first of all, the bathroom (which is what we usually do with guests

ATTITUDES AS THERAPY

in our homes) and explaining the location of equipment for personal hygiene. At this time, she may suggest that a bath or shower would help the patient feel better, and, if it is a routine, she will explain that and proceed with it, observing the patient for physical signs of previously attempted self-destruction, scars, illness, etc.

Her next explanation, which should follow immediately, will be that of the meal system operating in that hospital or ward. She should explain about tray service, the time of meals, and the availability or lack of availability of snacks in the dining room, canteen, or snack bar. She should describe the routines for obtaining small items such as toothbrushes, cosmetics, candy, etc.

The nurse probably will be checking the patient's weight, taking his temperature, and carrying out similar routine admission procedures while making these explanations. Since they will be in his room and personal effects will be used during this time, she can go on with an explanation of the hospital's regulations for care of cosmetics, jewelry, money, or other personal property, and reassure the patient by her attitude of friendly interest that his rights as an individual and his integrity will not be infringed upon. She can at this time explain about his room, or his bed in the ward, offer to show him the solarium or lounge, and take him out there and introduce him to other patients.

Nurse-Patient Relationship

At this time too, she should explain her relationship to him. This means she must have a clear understanding of that herself. She is the nurse who will be on this ward during such and such hours; there are other nurses and aides or orderlies who will be there also, from whom the patient can obtain information, help, and friendly companionship at any time. At a certain time she and the others will leave the ward, but another nurse or nurses will take their places; there will be other adjunctive personnel, and he will find someone at hand at any time of the day or night. The nurse will relay his messages to the doctor, make contacts with the doctor for him, and carry out the orders of his doctor in caring for him. This is reassuring to the patient, and, even though he may forget some of the information given him at this time, the initial attitude of helpfulness, reassurance, and making him feel at ease can do much to start him off "on the right track."

If at this time the patient asks questions which the nurse cannot or feels she should not answer, she can refer him to the doctor, saying he will see the patient very soon and may be able to answer his questions. She can add that she will try to answer as many questions as she can because she knows he must have a number of them. The patient will now feel that he has an ally, and that he will be protected from himself and from others who may threaten him. He may not express this, and may even appear gruff, disdainful, or knowing, but these full and complete explanations are necessary and should be given to him.

The nurse should also explain that certain laboratory tests are carried out on all persons admitted to the hospital, and she can tell him a little about the blood work, urinalysis, or other tests which may be done. Since most persons in any sort of hospital expect this, even though they know little if anything about it, such information is usually well received. The nurse can very well inquire here if the patient has ever been in a hospital before, and this opening gambit may provide her with much information about the patient, who will often proceed to tell her about himself, revealing, without being aware of it, much that will be useful. As much as is possible of this conversation and the patient's reactions should be recorded. It can prove invaluable in planning further care and treatment.

Psychiatric hospitals usually have a rather full program of social activities, ranging from occupational therapy, done at specified hours on the ward, to a very active routine of recreation and occupations carried on in other buildings or sections of the hospital. The nurse should mention this, and explain that the occupational therapist probably will call upon the patient to learn a little about his interests and help him find something in which he may participate. The doctor usually will order such activity, and the patient should be told this. Usually the occupational therapist receives word of new admissions within twenty-four hours after admission and will come to the floor to meet the patient and discuss the program with him. This is true of other therapists such as the recreational therapist, the librarian, and, often, the dietitian, but these persons should not see the patient too soon after his admission, as it would prove bewildering. There are other routines also, such as laboratory tests, and interviews with the doctor, social worker, and psychologist, which occur during the first week of admission. If ward movies or simple afternoon teas are routine, the nurse should explain the forthcoming activity and see that the patient attends, or she may assign this task to another patient. Much depends upon the social setting of the ward itself.

Whether it is a self-contained unit with its own schedules for activities or operates as the central point of activities, the ward is a unit, and the people in it make up a group. Sociologists tell us that any two or more people constitute a group within which certain action may be expected; that is, all of us take certain roles within the group, usually unconsciously. Those who are leaders soon begin to take over directing activities, and those who are followers wait for word from the leader. Within such a highly organized group as a psychiatric unit, the roles are assigned rather roughly with the nurse as leader, adjunctive workers as assistants, and patients as followers. There are individual roles within this rough over-all pattern, but the patient will expect all employees to be leaders of some sort. The nurse is often looked upon as a mother figure (in the army, many of the patients called their nurses "ward mama"), a person who will take care of one, feed one, ask questions about personal hygiene, and see that proper rest is obtained and that disputes among siblings are settled. It is rather a big role to be placed upon young women, but those who enter nursing seem to "feel" the need for being mothers and unconsciously act the part. In just such a way, many patients in any hospital will act infantile and in need of much attention. It is an age-old pattern of "acting out" deep emotions, and when we know this pattern we are better able to fit ourselves into the role expected of us.

The nurse, then, is the leader of the group within the ward. Her role is that of a mother or a hostess, and her primary duties are seeing to the comfort of those persons within her unit. This entails contacting other hospital personnel, but, because the patients know that a nurse is within call twenty-four hours a day, a large part of the responsibility for treatment falls upon her. Her helpers—aides, assistants, orderlies, etc.—fill the role of older sisters and brothers, to the patient. The patient may go to them with his problems, but all ward problems will go to the nurse, and she, in turn, will take up with the doctor, who is in the role of the father or top authoritative figure, those problems she cannot handle.

The patient will unconsciously put himself into the role of a small child, no matter how adult he may be or even if he is the president of a huge business concern. In the hospital he is a dependent sick person, in need of care and attention. Some people are able to accept this role with more pleasure than are others. It is rather nice to have a roof over one's head, a clean bed, regular meals, and someone to talk to at any time. If you have ever been ill, you know the pleasant "cared-for" feeling which accompanies being hospitalized. Those who are more dependent than others, persons who crave being cared for, may accept being a patient without any protest, but sometimes dependent persons will deny their dependency; that is, they do not like to feel they cannot get along totally alone, and often they are the patients who complain the most, who find fault with the food, with the attendants, or with the medications, and, in short, are the gripers in the group. It is as if by complaining they are telling the world, "You see, I really don't enjoy being dependent; I am really a strong person." Difficult as it may be, a matter-of-fact attitude is best toward such patients. Through countless centuries the sick have been given the role of dependent children and the nurse the role of a good mother, and, by maintaining such roles, we are able to help large numbers of sick persons.

SUGGESTED REFERENCES

Menninger, William C., "Psychiatric Treatment Designed to Meet Unconscious Needs, "*American Journal of Psychiatry,* **93**: 347–360, 1936.

Preston, George H., *Psychiatry for the Curious,* Rinehart & Company, New York, 1940.

Preston, George H., *The Substance of Mental Health,* Rinehart & Company, New York, 1943.

Render, Helena W., *Nurse-Patient Relationships in Psychiatry,* McGraw-Hill Book Company, Inc., New York, 1947, pp. 1–40.

CHAPTER 3

Some Safety Factors in Mental Hospitals

SAFETY IN ANY HOSPITAL means carrying out the care and treatment of patients within the hospital with a minimum of danger. In a psychiatric hospital the job is particularly difficult, because the patients are ambulatory and often have strange ideas which may result in injury to others or to themselves. Each hospital will have its own safety rules, dependent upon the construction of the buildings and the problems presented therein. All safety rules are carefully planned to cover any contingency and should be followed to the letter. The safety of the patients is the prime responsibility of all personnel working in psychiatric hospitals.

While certain precautions are necessary to minimize danger, the best tools are knowledge and awareness of what the dangers may be. We cannot possibly remove all the objects with which persons may damage themselves or others. Hence, we must be constantly alert to the least sign that something is wrong. It may be no more than a feeling that a certain patient is going to "explode," or it may be a thin curl of smoke coming from the broom closet. To know what to do and how to do it is the direct responsibility of every person working in the psychiatric hospital.

Two great hazards stand out above all others—suicide and fire. The prevention of suicide is a constant concern; the employee who picks up a bit of broken glass lying on the lawn or finds the hidden corset string in a patient's bedding may have prevented a suicide. We can never tell how often we prevent suicide; our job is to continue the daily, undramatic, watchful care of those in our charge.

Fire is the other frightening hazard, and every employee must know the location of fire extinguishers and what to do in case of a blaze. Fire drills may seem dull, but the routines must be mastered so thoroughly that each step will be executed automatically in the event of a real fire.

Safety includes, too, protection of patients from their fellows who are so ill as to be combative and destructive, and protection of such patients from themselves. Alertness as to the whereabouts of all patients at all times is the first rule of safety.

Use of Equipment

Next, we must know what the patients are doing, what tools and equipment they are using in the course of their work in occupational therapy or industrial therapy, and if those tools or equipment are where others may get to them. Seriously disturbed and disoriented patients should never have access to knives, scissors, carpentry tools, or even such innocuous-appearing instruments as knitting needles or crochet hooks. It is wise to have the latter equipment made of plastic, though this too can be dangerous. The ordinary tools of dining can be used as destructive weapons by disturbed patients, but with modern plastics and paper equipment an attractive and nondangerous tray or table setting can be made. In removing the injurious equipment, every effort must be made to keep living conditions pleasant and as normal in appearance as possible. The self-respect of patients can be maintained by the use of attractive paper or plastic materials utilized matter-of-factly. Many patients are so in the habit of using table silver that, even though they are disturbed, it is a good idea to have them continue using it. Close observance is all that is necessary, and a silver count is the usual thing in all psychiatric hospitals. This need need not be so obvious that it is irritating to patients. All persons helping with the serving of food should familiarize themselves with the amount of silver on hand and the amount used at each meal, and should be able to see at a glance when a utensil is missing. Each hospital has its own method of checking equipment, but a check at the end of each meal is the rule, and missing articles mean an *immediate* search.

Often, patients will hide a piece of silver just to see the excitement caused when its loss is discovered. Searches should be calm, quiet, and without a punitive attitude. Should equipment still be missing after the immediate search, the loss must be reported to someone in authority; responsibility for further search will be taken by that person. Favorite hiding places are in window frames and doorframes, under the tables and chairs in the supporting crossbars, or on the patient's person. If it is necessary to search the patients themselves, try to maintain dignity and apologize for the need to search. An attitude such as this often discourages further attempts. The disapproval of fellow patients will also discourage the patient from making such attention-getting efforts. Use of table silver to make keys or weapons for self-destruction must be kept in mind always, but such use must never be mentioned to the patients. Discussions among the patients about this should be discouraged by a tactful changing of the subject.

Keys are a great source of difficulty in psychiatric hospitals, and it is wise to recognize just what the keys may signify. Many persons are afraid of being in a locked room or building, but more important than that is the affront to the freedom and dignity of the person. Even a patient who has no desire to leave a room is angered by the knowledge that he cannot leave should he so desire. The keys represent authority in those who handle them and, like all authority, should be carried quietly and without great show. It is rude as well as unwise to jangle the keys unnecessarily, make comments about them, or carry them with a great fuss. Carrying keys on heavy chains ostentatiously jangling at the waist is as unnecessary as it is unwise. Whenever possible, locks should be one of a kind on all doors so that only one or two keys need

SOME SAFETY FACTORS IN MENTAL HOSPITALS

be carried by personnel. These can be kept in a pocket where they are easily available to the person carrying them but out of reach of patients. All personnel should carry a restraint key with the master key. In an emergency much time can be lost looking for a restraint key if only one person carries it. Medicine-cupboard keys should be carried only by the nurses, and all medicine cupboards should be kept locked at all times when they are not in use.

Linen cupboards and closets for cleaning equipment should also be kept locked to cut down the hazard of patients' hiding in them or hiding harmful objects in them. Patients' clothing cupboards are usually kept locked in buildings housing disturbed patients, but they may be opened at the patient's request to get an article of clothing. At this time, someone must remain with the patient to see what is taken out and to lock up after use. Such items as belts, neckties, extra shoelaces, and corset strings are usually counted and, in some hospitals, kept in the nurse's service station to ensure closer observation of such obviously good material for hanging. Nurses and attendants often become impatient at the amount of personal equipment which can be dangerous, but simple checking systems are easily set up, depending on the construction of the ward, and patients will readily fall into the customs of the ward in which they are living. It is fairly common practice to lock cosmetics cupboards. Wooden drawers or trays with a slot for a patient's name card help keep items separated, and all personnel should familiarize themselves with the equipment belonging to each patient. An original check list is kept with the patient's chart, and any new equipment brought or sent to the patient must be added to that list. Any equipment disposed of should be checked off the list to prevent unnecessary searching.

A cosmetics check-out list is used by some hospitals; in others a member of the nursing staff is assigned to cosmetic checking for the day and will keep track of what has been issued and check it in at night.

Items commonly checked in and counted are the following:

- Artificial dentures
- Artificial limbs or appliances of any kind
- Belts
- Cleansing creams
- Clippers
- Cologne
- Cigarette lighters
- Sanitary belts
- Tweezers
- Eyeglasses
- Hairpins
- Hair tonic
- Inexpensive jewelry
- Ink
- Knitting and crocheting equipment
- Scissors
- Tooth paste
- Lotions
- Needles and pins
- Personal medications
- Nail files
- Pictures in metal frames with glass
- Razors (see next paragraph)
- Suspenders
- Watches and clocks

Many hospitals will not allow razors in any locked building; either a barber and beautician are available, or shaving is done at specified hours under close supervision with a special razor. Some hospitals allow only electric razors to be used. Care must be taken that the bathroom outlet for electric razors is far enough from sinks, tubs, and toilets so patients cannot plug in equipment and make contact with the water pipes or water. Even with an electric razor, shaving is done under supervision because of the danger of the patient's using the cord to hang himself, and even in unlocked wards a careful razor check is made; if safety razors are used, a count must be made of blades. Dangerous articles may be used by other patients as well as by the one checking them out.

No mention has been made of matches because, almost uniformly, patients are forbidden to use them at any time. In most hospitals all personnel carry matches to light cigarettes for patients. It has been found useful in some hospitals to have cigarette lighters on all floors, to suggest that all personnel carry only lighters and no matches, and to allow less disturbed patients to have their own lighters, which are marked with their names and checked in and out like other items of personal property. Matches will be brought in by visitors, or, if patients obtain cigarettes from a vending machine, matches usually come with them, as do a couple of pennies change. This should be checked in some manner. While the individual patient may be perfectly able to handle them, matches are such common household items that people tend to be careless with them, and less capable persons may pick them up. Bad hospital fires have been started by patients and are a constant danger.

Restraints

Types and Uses. Discussion of restraint has been put off until last because there is so much misuse of it, as well as misunderstanding of what restraint actually is. The dictionary tells us that restraint means to hold from action, or to limit. We use many forms of restraint, and the use of terms other than restraint does not change the purpose or intent of the act itself. All of us are familiar with the restraining word or gesture used with a child about to do something which has been forbidden. Mother's head-shaking and use of "No, no" is a form of restraint, as it limits the action of the child (usually). Some psychiatrists tell us that the conscience or superego is the mother shaking her head "no."

Much of the time, sensitivity to patient reactions can make the use of restraint unnecessary. Diverting activity before it reaches a level needing restraint is one of the nurse's simplest and best methods of meeting the moral and legal problem of restraint.

Nonetheless, much as we like to feel we don't "restrain" patients, it is a pretty common practice. The use of locked buildings or wards is a form of restraint, as is the system of liberties utilized in some hospitals. By withholding a special privilege, such as attending a movie, we limit the patient's actions to meet our demands. Medication is a frequent, unhappily a too frequent, form of restraint. All too often a nurse gives sedatives to relieve herself of the challenge and irritation of the patient who is demanding. It is so simple to keep him quiet and to rationalize by saying, "He needs a rest." Actually, in such cases, we are saying, "I can't stand his constant questions, or his sitting up past 'lights out.'" If we face honestly the use of restraints, and ask ourselves why we are giving medications, withholding privileges, or refusing requests, we can then meet the problems of the destructive and overactive patient more objectively. Restraints are necessary, and we do use them.

What are some of the types of restraint used? They vary from hospital to hospital and state to state. Some hospitals use the leather wristband and anklet with the leather strap which is fastened to the bed. Less common today but still used all too frequently are the restraint jacket or strait jacket, the humane sheet, and the muff. Occasionally, all types of reasoning fail to capture the patient's attention or allow us to help him. Then, until he can be reached, it is necessary to apply some form of mechanical or chemical restraint.

It is wise to know the laws of the state in which you are nursing before applying any form of restraint. All new employees should familiarize themselves first with the laws and then with the hospital rules. If the hospital's rules are contrary to the state law, it is your duty to refuse to carry out the act and to point out why you are refusing. The law, however, usually states that, in an emergency, the person acting in the capacity of a nurse or doctor must do whatever a reasonable man would do in a like situation. It is wise to remember that the law specifies that the act must be reasonable. Strait jackets and chains do not appear reasonable under any circumstances.

Hydrotherapy in many forms is a method of restraining, particularly in such forms as continuous tub baths and wet-sheet pack. Properly given and with a cheerful, matter-of-fact, helpful attitude, either bath or pack may prove pleasant and most helpful.

Attitudes in the Use of Restraint. Restraint should be used only when necessary, upon written order of the physician, and as a form of treatment. Punitive attitudes are unwise in the application of restraint of any kind since they create antagonism on the part of the patient, which, in turn, brings out antagonism in the person applying them. Since the use of restraint often means the use of extra help, it is wise to be sure there is enough help on hand to work together, and to work quietly, quickly, and calmly. All persons who will be required to use any form of restraint should know the method used by the hospital where they are employed so there will be smooth, simplified action in an emergency.

It is not at all amiss to apologize for putting a patient in restraint and to promise to remove it as soon as the patient is better able to handle his emotions. The promise should, of course, be kept. Patients approached in this manner soon realize that restraint is not punishment but a method of helping them to control or limit actions which have got out of their own immediate control. Many patients recognize this and will ask to be put in restraint before they "hurt somebody." This approach is so successful that nurses sometimes can put patients in restraint without the aid of a large number of assistants, and often a patient will help get his pack bed ready. To use a punitive attitude will only provoke behavior intended to annoy the mother figure; this builds up guilt in the patient and results in his needing more punishment. Hence, it is much wiser to use the attitude of applying restraint, in any form, as a treatment which can and will be changed when the patient is better able to control himself or the situation in which he finds himself.

Attitudes as a Form of Restraint. We all react to the attitudes of others, sometimes without being consciously aware of the reaction. Patients are more sensitive to our attitudes than we are to theirs, partly because they seem to have a more acute sensitivity, and partly because they are quite watchful of us. Theirs is a rather narrow world in the hospital, and they get to know it and its boundaries quite well. We can utilize this trait of patients in their care. Often a first step to recovery is taken by the patient who will do something for a particular nurse or attendant. While this can be and is a useful tool, it should not so flatter the nurse thus successful to the point where she exploits it, because this will result in injury to the patient's self-esteem and a dangerous dependence on the nurse or attendant. Since patients generally do like the approval of the nursing and attendant staff, however, and can readily sense disapproval of their acts, this is a useful tool in meeting such asocial behavior as rudeness in a group, squabbling, and minor social offenses.

The irritation or hostility of the group itself can sometimes hinder further asocial behavior, but sometimes it acts as a means to spur the patient on to even greater misbehavior in an effort to retain the attention of the group. With the doctor's permission, it may be necessary to point out to the patient that there are more socially acceptable ways of getting attention, or it may be necessary to remove him from the group, telling him he may return when his behavior is more acceptable. Your own attitude of nonacceptance and disapproval will get across to the patient without your making a great effort to let him see that you disapprove. Most persons stand in such great need of the approval of others that your attitude and that of the group will act effectively as restraint. It is a useful tool to keep on hand, especially as those patients who expect and hope to return to normal life will find the group in their normal social world less accepting of misbehavior than the group in the hospital.

In the dining room a patient may be messy with his food, mixing everything together or eating untidily. The nurse can suggest quietly that it is unpleasant to eat with someone who acts this way, and either imply or say outright that such a person will have to eat alone until his eating habits meet group standards. Conversation should be acceptable too, and the nurse should have enough small talk at her command to keep mealtime conversation at a light, agreeable level. It is quite acceptable for the nurse to say quietly, "That's not very good table conversation," if talk becomes distressing. It is equally acceptable to say, "What a morbid discussion," or, "Let's talk about something else," in any group where conversation appears to be reaching a point leading to overstimulation or morbidity.

Ability to restrain by use of conversation is a rather special skill, but a nurse can prepare for this without being a social leader by keeping up with the news, sports, or theater. A beginner might keep a newspaper handy, or bring in a clever cartoon, or mention one she knows the group has seen in the current periodicals. Very simple conversational gambits are a good means of starting group activity such as a lively discussion. This may not appear to be restraint, but in its promotion of desirable social behavior, good conversation is quite a useful restraining technique. Antisocial behavior is sometimes a reaction to boredom in the hospital. Even without an active occupational therapy program, a group can be guided away from boredom by lively conversation. It is the most natural form of activity at anyone's command, and probably the least expensive treatment as well as the most available.

SUGGESTED REFERENCES

Erickson, Isabel, "The Nursing Problems in the Psychiatric Hospital," *Hospitals*, 11:58–62, 1937.

Mathenay, R. V., and Topelis, M., "Nursing Care for the Acutely Ill Psychotic Patient," *American Journal of Nursing*, 50:27–29, 1950.

Patten, Edith, "Psychiatric Nursing in the General Hospital," *American Journal of Nursing*, 45:193–195, 1945.

Weiss, Madeline O., "Attempted Suicide—Then What?" *American Journal of Nursing*, 49:290, 1949.

CHAPTER 4

The Art of Answering Questions

WHY DO SOME OF US dislike to answer questions? Why do we hate taking tests? Usually, because we don't know the answers to the questions or are so insecure about our knowledge that we become frightened. Nurses are asked many questions throughout the hospital day. Some of these are foolish-sounding, some are serious and worried questions, and some are merely attention-getting mechanisms. All should be answered, and the nurse should be so secure in her work, so sure of her own limitations, that questions do not trouble her. If she feels secure in her work, if she truly likes her job, she will not mind answering questions, nor will she mind admitting it if she doesn't know the answer.

The first step toward such security is the recognition that questioners do not always expect the person questioned to know the answer. In fact, the person who does know all the answers becomes a rather threatening, awesome creature, not nearly so well liked as the happy-go-lucky person who can give a ready and untroubled, "I don't know, but I'll try to find out." Self-assurance does not necessitate knowing all the answers, or even appearing as if one knows them; it entails only being comfortable with one's self and not trying to live up to impossible standards. Usually we are our own hardest taskmasters, and, as we set standards more difficult to reach, our assurance falls lower and lower. The nurse is taught a tremendous amount of material in a very short time, and it is not expected that she will remember all she has been taught.

Formal education teaches the sources of materials and how to use those sources. The rest is up to the individual. Some persons have a more retentive memory than others, but it is of greater importance to remember where we can find material in the library or which doctor will be most willing and able to assist one to find an answer than to try to memorize facts. No one nurse could possibly foresee what questions will be asked by every patient, so the impossible task of storing knowledge to answer all questions is best ignored. The next best thing is to be willing to say you don't know, calmly and without being defensive or apologetic. This is a sign of assurance, of knowing yourself well enough not to apologize because you have met a new situation for which you are not totally prepared. Often the question itself is not so important to the patient as is the attitude you will take in replying to it.

What Patients' Questions Mean

Why do patients ask questions, especially if they don't really expect an answer? First of all, when we are insecure we look about us, question everything we see, and try to familiarize ourselves with everything within our reach. That is what many patients do by asking questions. They are actually saying, "I am insecure and frightened. I don't know what to expect, and the unknown is most fearful." A hospital can be a very frightening place to a lay person, and we can realize this if we recall our early student days and the fright and awe we felt about places, equipment, and scientific names which are now so much a part of our lives that we think nothing of them. Familiarity, after long days of careful instruction, led to this security, and we cannot expect a sick person to get the "feel" of a hospital rapidly. The sick person has many problems other than his immediate illness, or complicating his immediate illness, and we must expect him to be insecure. Because of this, the patient will want to test those around him. He will want to see if he stands alone in this feeling, or if the personnel, too, are insecure and unknowing and frightened. He will want to see if he is the authority figure or if the nurse is. This is called testing; it is something all children do as they grow up and learn what they may and may not do safely.

Human beings differ from other animals in their ability to recall and formulate abstract ideas; hence, many of the safety rules of living are a part of our unconscious lives, and we react without conscious thought. The sick person becomes rather like a small child learning anew. His ability to recall may be hampered by distracting thoughts or sights or sounds. He may be distorting reality, and he must test, and test again, often by asking questions, and often by asking the same questions again and again. Or he may be merely testing your patience to see how far he may go with you, and how long you can hold out. When this is suspected, it is perfectly normal to remind the patient that you have answered that same question many times, and ask him why he repeats it.

We have mentioned testing reality; this is most important to the patient who is living in a frightening world where he feels threatened by the insecurity of not knowing what is real and what is not real. He may ask questions because reality is just beyond his grasp, and it will take endless patience and kindness to get him to accept reality for what it is. His unreal world may mean more to him than the reality of rising, bathing, and mingling with strangers in a locked building. The least hint of laughing at him and at his questions, or at his peculiarities, may cause him to withdraw into the unreal world of his fantasies, where he can make his characters like him, and, most important, not laugh at him. Let him test reality constantly, but don't play with the unreality of his fantasies, tease him, or question him about them. It may be simpler to evade his questions, or to be annoyed and hasty with him, but the most important thing to remember is that, when he is testing reality, it is your responsibility to make reality a thing he will welcome and be able to accept. Repeat, and repeat again if necessary, but guide him to the actual world in which he exists.

Sometimes the questions are rather ridiculous, and the

THE ART OF ANSWERING QUESTIONS

nurse will have to judge for herself, as she gains security and knowledge in this field, whether or not the patient is truly testing reality or is just trying to gain attention. We usually can recognize the attention-getting questions. All of us are familiar with the student who always asks questions in class, the person who always asks questions of the visiting lecturer, or the person who interrupts a story. This is undoubtedly attention-getting. It must be handled skillfully in order not to embarrass the person but to guide him to seek attention in some other more socially acceptable manner.

There are certain methods of answering questions which everyone should know, as they prove helpful in daily living as well as in the hospital. Much of how we answer depends on the first two subjects mentioned earlier, self-assurance or inner security, and what the questions mean.

Answering Questions by Asking a Question

This method is old but effective and proves extremely useful in social situations where one doesn't care to answer a direct question or is embarrassed by it, as well as when it is inadvisable to give a direct answer to a patient.

Perhaps the patient will ask, "Do you think I'm crazy?" This can be met with several questions: "What makes you ask that?" "Do you think you're crazy?" "What do you mean by crazy?" Any one of these answers avoids a direct "yes" or "no" reply and will lead to further talk which may be helpful to the patient. Answers to "Why doesn't the doctor let me go into town?" "When am I going to go home?" "Will they ever let me out of here?" "What is that medicine?" ad infinitum can be met with the question, "Have you discussed that with your doctor?" or "Why don't you ask the doctor when he comes around?" Many questions can be met pleasantly and jocularly, depending on the patient, and that is something which each nurse learns for herself as she gets the "feel" of patient attitudes, for example: "Now what on earth made you think of that?" "Why do you ask me all these questions?" "How do you manage to think of so many questions?"

"Do you think you could go into town alone?" "Are you fearful of the medication?" "Why don't you want the medicine (or treatment)?"

As you work with patients daily, you will learn the best method of asking a question when asked one, often merely taking the patient's question and turning it into a questioning answer. Other questions and other patients require different types of answers, and these again depend on familiarity with the field and the patients under your care.

Direct Answers

Strangely enough, direct answers seem to be the most difficult for people to make, and nurses often become evasive and defensive in many cases where a simple, straightforward answer would serve the purpose well. Perhaps we must practice saying "yes" and "no" without putting too much emotional tone into it, for a calm "no" will often prove most effectual in quieting a disturbed person's fearful and provocative questions, as will an equally calm "yes."

This brings up the use of such flat answers in meeting amorous patients' advances. Often patients will ask you to kiss them, and a calm, quiet "no" will prove quite effective in stopping further advances or requests. Should the patient ask you why, you can then answer by saying, "Why do you ask me to kiss you?" to which the patient may very well reply that you are attractive or look like his wife or sweetheart. At that point you can lead up to the fact that you are a nurse and he (or she) is a patient, and by this time, the general idea of refusal and professional relationships is pretty much put across. It is difficult to meet amorous advances without being coy or provocative—a perfectly normal response from anyone—but matter-of-fact, direct answers can save both you and the patient from embarrassing tussles, and it is wise to remember that, on recovery, many patients are quite embarrassed by the behavior they exhibited while ill.

Since too often there is no amnesia for many of the things patients say or do while disturbed, if they can look back on such a period and recall that it was met with kindness and calm, they feel little or no guilt and no need to be a bit defensive with you.

Obscene language and requests also can be met with direct answers, followed by the suggestion to change to more moderate language even in expressing anger. The nurse must not express any disgust or irritation when making such suggestions, as this provokes further attempts to arouse her. Patients are very like children, whose outbursts are as much to get attention as to release inner tensions. Often the best approach is to ignore such outbursts, unless they come at a time and place where a quiet, firm reminder of the basic social amenities is useful.

Referral to Other Sources

This has been discussed briefly in meeting questions by answering with such a reply as, "Have you taken that up with your doctor?" but it can be extended to acknowledgment of the nurse's not knowing the answer and a suggestion to ask someone who does, depending on the question and who would know the answer.

Referral can be made to many sources, both persons and books, and often this is an opportunity to introduce new personnel to the patient—personnel who may be of help in the patient's hospital stay or rehabilitation. Thus, a question about cost of hospitalization may be referred to the social worker, who may have had no call to see the patient until now, or whom the patient may have refused to see until now. Questions about food may be referred to the dietitian, and it is a good idea for the dietitian to meet all new patients whenever that is possible. Many questions can be referred to the doctor, to another nurse who has some knowledge of the special point that has been raised, to an occupational therapist, recreational therapist, or librarian. From this a new hobby may be started, or an old one revived. Referral to other sources can be an opening gambit which will lead to remarkable socialization of the patient who has heretofore kept much to himself. If it is possible to refer the patient to another patient who has worked with a subject about which the first has asked, this too is good, for now two patients benefit. There seem to be no limits to where referral can lead, and again it points up how important it is for the nurse to know not all the answers but some of the sources of answers.

Offering Help in Getting Answers

This follows closely referral to other sources, as the patient may be too shy or too frightened and bewildered to make any effort other than to ask a question. The nurse can help by offering to get the referred source, or in some way making it available. She may even ask the question of someone else and come back with the answer, adding that she got the answer from such and such a person. Then, when the patient meets this person there is a small but common point of interest to start him toward socializing. If the question can be answered by finding a book, the nurse may stop in the library and get the book for the patient. The librarian may not be needed at this point, but if the patient does not return the book this is a good time for the librarian to come to get it, and another meeting, which may have been awkward otherwise, fits in with the pattern of hospital life.

All these points about answering questions may appear unimportant, but they can uncover many interesting facts about the patient, his background, and his plans for recovery, which are useful tools in psychiatry, and they emphasize, too, that one of the most important arts in nursing is that of being a good hostess. The words "hostess" and "hospital" actually come from the same source, which means literally "to protect the stranger." In nursing we should accept the fact that we are protecting the patient not only from disease organisms but from social sources of irritation and difficulty. It takes skill and interest to be a truly good nurse or hostess, but one can take pride in work well done and a deep sense of satisfaction in seeing a disturbed and frightened person well enough to go home, or even well enough to mingle socially in a group of patients and employees. That is why answering questions is called an art. Nursing is in itself an art of the highest order, requiring skill in many things besides making a bed, giving a bath, pouring medications, and applying dressings.

SUGGESTED REFERENCE

Guide to the Order Sheet (mimeographed pamphlet), The Menninger Foundation, Topeka, Kans., 1946, pp. 26–29.

CHAPTER 5

General Attitudes Used

For someone trying to explain anything as intangible as attitudes, the *Dictionary of Psychology,* by Howard C. Warren of Princeton University, is an excellent book. This book says that an attitude is "the specific mental disposition toward an incoming (or arising) experience, whereby that experience is modified, or a condition of readiness for a certain activity." We use the term "professionalism" as a general synonym for the attitudes taken toward patients. In that cover-all term is implied a mixture of objectivity, friendliness, and sympathy. In psychiatry we sometimes use the word "empathy" in place of "sympathy," and the meanings are similar. Sympathy is defined as a fellow feeling, a relationship between things so that whatever affects one similarly affects the other, or a mutual susceptibility. Empathy is said to be the projection of one's own consciousness into another being, or an identification with another. We use both sympathy and empathy fairly unconsciously, but, made aware of these feelings, we can utilize the emotions arising from our contacts with patients to help them recover a more normal state. This may be the basis of whatever it is which makes a "good" psychiatric nurse.

No two persons have exactly the same mental make-up, which helps make life more interesting while adding to its more complicated pattern. With little conscious effort on our part, our general attitude is what makes us take up nursing, and later the special branch of nursing in which we earn our

Security and Protection

Safety devices and other mechanical means are not the only ways of protecting the patient. Security and protection may also come in a large measure from attitudes. We mentioned in a previous chapter that our own attitudes can do much to make a patient feel secure and protected. How does that work? A patient may enter the hospital filled with fears for his own safety, or for the safety of his family, and we can help him by matter-of-factly explaining the ward situation in which he will live, answering his questions, referring him to other sources for help, and being there when he needs us. Just as a child feels secure when he knows he is in the same room with his mother, the patient feels secure knowing that a nurse is within sight of him throughout the twenty-four hours. That is one reason nurses work the clock around. Often a patient may not need any physical care during the night, but he is reassured knowing that a nurse is at her desk and may be reached by light, buzzer, or merely by calling. He feels he may sleep because someone who is interested in him, whose only job is interest in him and his fellows, is right there where she can be reached. This is really protection. Our constant presence plus our understanding and easy availability then give the patient a feeling of security and protection. He may question this at first and may use the ruses he used as a child—wanting a drink of water, wanting to go to the bathroom, crying out, or complaining of pain. Children do the same thing, not to see how often mother will come without scolding when called but to be sure mother really is there when he calls.

Perhaps this is a good place to explain why I say patients

are often like small children. When people become ill, they often discard adult standards of behavior, partly because of pain and fear and partly because illness often simulates a return to childhood in which physical care by a mother figure, reliance on a nurse and doctor for important decisions, and routines of bathing, meals, and sleep—similar to a child's—are controlled fairly rigidly, as most childhood routines are. This regression to a childhood pattern is often useful while the patient is acutely ill. There is a danger point in it for the patient, who may so like to be directed and cared for that it is difficult to get him to accept again the more independent adult status. (Usually this is unconscious, as are most of our real feelings.) The danger point for the nurse is her own satisfaction in managing or manipulating the life of another, so that she is unwilling to see the patient regain health and more mature behavior. The psychiatric nurse must be on guard for these danger points, and use of attitudes as therapy is helpful in facing the problems as they arise and in handling them skillfully and satisfactorily for the good of society.

I have mentioned earlier that restraint may be a form of protection, giving the patient a feeling of security. Because of our upbringing, most of us feel it is wrong to voice hostility, or do aggressive and hostile things such as smashing china, swearing, etc. In the psychiatric patient, his need to express hostility is stronger than his training, and he will do many things that he would not do ordinarily. In fact, he may be ill because he restrained himself *from* expressing hostility. Once in a hospital he can say what he pleases, break things, and be pretty abusive. Personnel who understand him are all about, and while they may guide him to more acceptable ways of expressing his hostility, they are not shocked, nor do they scold or punish. More important, they are not members of his family, with all the intermingled emotions of love and hatred, so they cannot be hurt by what he says and does. This gives him a feeling of security; he may say and do hostile things to these strangers (who act as a substitute family), but, in so doing, he is secure in the affection of his family because they do not bear the brunt of his hostility. Since hostility is often felt toward those near and dear to us, while we continue to love them, he may feel he wishes to harm the members of his family or his close associates. In the hospital he will be prevented from doing so, and thus he feels protected. When he is able to discuss his hostile acts and feelings with the doctor, he will not have as great accompanying guilt for them as if he had said and done those hostile things in his home, and hence will be better able to discuss them objectively. He will see other patients around him with the same sort of behavior, the same repressed rage and fear, and he will find that he is not alone in his mixed feelings and bewildering emotions. This, too, will give him a feeling of security, for when we are not alone in what we do, we can feel more confident.

The use of mechanical restraint, although not the best method of treating the mentally ill, is necessary occasionally. When used properly and with the attitude of helping the patient over a difficult period while he is unable to control his reactions, it will result in a strong feeling of protection and security. In a way, it is as if the patient thinks, "These people will not let me injure others or myself. They will see to it that I don't hurt those I love in any way, and they will not punish me." Indeed, some patients will ask for that type of protection. Sometimes, patients will say and do very unpleasant things and will accuse the personnel of putting up with them only because they are paid to do so. It is wise to agree at this point, but to add that there are many other jobs in the world, and you chose that of helping the mentally ill because you like and are interested in people. It is true you are paid for being "nice" to patients who are not always nice in return, but if the work didn't interest you, you wouldn't remain in the position. This, too, is reassuring and protective, and if said with true feeling, the patient will again get the idea that you are there to help him, and he will respond to that helpfulness.

Helpfulness

Here is another attitude which is general and rather vague, and we must stop to consider just how we can be helpful without "spoon-feeding" the ill. Sometimes, indeed, we are most helpful when we insist rigidly on the patient's standing alone and figuring things out for himself. The dictionary tells us that helpfulness is the relieving of pain or disease, being useful. With this meaning in mind, we can approach the attitude somewhat differently and examine what we do more carefully. Nurses like to believe they are helpful people, naturally. Sometimes we get so involved in our own ideas of being a lady with a lamp that we are helpful when people would just as soon we weren't. In psychiatry it is a particularly delicate task to maintain an attitude of being helpful when you must deny the patient many of the amenities of his normal living. Sometimes the doctors' orders seem strange and even cruel—such as not permitting the patient to see his family, or to make a telephone call—and it is at such times that it is wise to recall that helpfulness means mitigating a disease. The doctor must have some very good reason for his order, so you must follow it to the letter, but explain the patient's reaction carefully on his chart. Be sure your own reaction is one of friendly interest, but carry out the doctor's order, no matter how unpleasant.

Acutely disturbed and hallucinatory patients may be hindered by family visits because of an inability to recognize visitors, or because the patient may be so delusional that the visit forces him into further flight from reality. The patient may feel that the visitors are plotting against him, attempting to kill him, or have placed him in the hospital in order to get his money. The visitors naturally are distressed by these ideas in a loved one and will often argue, wheedle, or cajole the patient in an effort to change him. Because we cannot change delusions or hallucinations by willing them to be changed, visits are often a hindrance to recovery. While visits are forbidden or restricted to very limited periods, the doctor and staff are working toward the goal of getting the patient back into reality, and many hospitals have social workers who keep in touch with the family and endeavor to help them understand the illness and how they may assist in the patient's recovery. In those cases where ancillary workers are few and the nurse is the contact with the patient's family, it is wise for her to discuss visitor and patient reactions with the doctor and make appointments for the family to see the doctor so that they may discuss the current regulations.

Delusional patients also may attempt to make phone calls or write letters which can precipitate uncomfortable situations or complicated legal battles. They may become obscene or threatening, and no one is well served if such calls and letters are allowed to reach the public. The doctor often is more fully aware of these facts about individual patients than is the nurse, and he has them in mind when he writes orders which may appear very rigid or limiting. *We cannot compromise with anyone and continue being helpful.*

We must be ready at all times to assist the patient in whatever way is best for his recovery, remaining within the limits of the orders of the physician and continuing to let the patient know we are friendly and available for assistance. It is well to be able to converse freely and easily on a broad number of subjects, to have a working knowledge of many of the arts and crafts he will be occupied with in the hospital, to be able to play simple card games and take part in other simple sports, to be able to attend a dance or theater with him, to be socially pleasant but professional, and to recognize at all times that he is a patient and you are a nurse—a paid professional whose job it is to help this person return to his role in society.

Permissiveness

This attitude is sometimes called being nonjudgmental, and it is always a problem in group management because patients will react with annoyance or petulance to seeing another patient doing things or breaking some minor rule which they themselves may not be permitted to do. Permissiveness must be administered judiciously, on the order of the physician, and must not be based on the nurse's personal feelings toward the patient. It is rather easy to fall into the trap of being permissive with a particularly appealing patient, and this may be just the patient who has attempted to get by throughout his life on his appeal. His failure to do so in a mature society is just what got him in the hospital, and the nurse who reacts to his personality by permissiveness is delaying his recovery. Such persons have to learn that there are times when a code of behavior must be rather rigidly adhered to, and that personal charm will not excuse them. It is such patients who will play one nurse against the other, the nurse against the doctor, and patients against the nurse. Hence it is necessary to put aside personal feelings while on duty and follow the attitudes ordered throughout the entire day and night. Difficult as it is to refrain from permissiveness to some patients of charm, it is even more difficult to be permissive to patients who do not show much charm or affability, but for whom this attitude is ordered. These persons need to learn that they may break an occasional rule, that minor infractions will not result in their being ostracized, and that the world will not collapse about them if they tell a little falsehood. Often persons for whom permissiveness is ordered are afflicted with an overactive conscience, expecting too much of themselves as well as others, and are unable to meet their high expectations; or they may be persons too withdrawn and unaware of reality to know what rules and regulations keep their particular group cohesive. Permissiveness may range from allowing such a patient to sit up past bedtime (even all night, occasionally) to getting special foods for him, to overlooking his returning from town late on pass. Certain very rigid rules of all hospitals are not overlooked for these patients or any others, of course. These are the regulations about no matches, not allowing a patient to handle keys *at any time,* keeping certain doors and windows locked, and similar safety rules. Permissiveness for the individual patient never encroaches upon the safety of the group.

GENERAL ATTITUDES USED

Permissiveness often is given to patients in the routines of daily care. Such a person may want to be the first to bathe, or the last to be served his food, or he may want special foods, to read books not allowed other patients, or to sit by the nurse's desk when it is time to go to bed. With the doctor's help, the nurse may make arrangements to fit these idiosyncrasies into the scheduled nursing care. She may have to contact the family or dietitian for certain foods and the librarian for the books or magazines he wants, or she may have to recognize that his sitting by her desk reading at eleven at night is perfectly all right. Her routines may be disarranged for a short time, but the patient will gain so greatly in his trust of nurses and hospital personnel that his therapy will be more acceptable to him. Patients are individuals, and when a person becomes sick, he will cling to many little things from his past in an effort to retain his individuality, which is often threatened by the group regulations. We can build his shaky faith in us with permissiveness until he can learn to meet the greater demands of group membership and no longer needs a special atmosphere.

Matter-of-factness

A matter-of-fact attitude is like a boat's anchor in stormy waters. The boat may bob about, become submerged, or be flooded, but it is held to one spot until the storm blows over. All of us know at least one person to whom we turn in moments of distress because that person is so calm and accepting of events, so matter-of-fact, that what we thought unsolvable soon becomes a simple problem easily met. This is really an ability to view objectively the situation at the moment and still be able to keep the end goal in view. Actually, we must use it pretty routinely in general nursing care, as when we enter a patient's room and say, "It's time for your bath." There is no question about the patient's wanting a bath or setting any special time for the bath. This is it, and we proceed. Of course, such an attitude is not so simple when the patient is querulous or argumentative, and the nurse must be tactful and pleasant in using such an approach. Brusqueness is a danger point the nurse must guard against in using this attitude. In carrying out care and treatment, we must avoid challenging the patient or allowing the least doubt to creep into our action. We must not fall into the sometimes enjoyable trap of arguing or becoming defensive with the patient. His irritability or distrust can be met with the suggestion that the questioned matter be discussed with his doctor, but at the moment we shall carry on with the procedure ordered. Interestingly, although patients may fuss and complain about the matter-of-fact person, or about the staff's seeming rigidity, they often will cling to that very person or the rigid routine, when they are disturbed.

Kind Firmness

There is a fine boundary line between matter-of-factness and firmness which is difficult to define. Indeed, one may say firmness is a bit brusque, though never unkind. Here is rigidity despite protestations of despair and anger, and the nurse implies or even tells the patient she will accept no deviation from the rule. She expects certain duties, routines, and tasks to be done, and she gives sparingly of praise for performance, though she does not fail to thank the patient if it is indicated. This depends upon how firm the doctor wishes the staff to be. Often, in ordering a firm attitude, the doctor asks that the patient be assigned simple menial tasks such as helping serve trays, emptying ash trays, cleaning up the bathrooms, pulling weeds, etc. These are tasks assigned to help the patient recover rather than to aid the hospital staff, which means that thanks and praise do not fit into carrying out the attitude. Should a patient assigned this attitude perform a little act of courtesy such as opening a door for you or helping you with your coat, thanks are expected and should be given. The firmness applies to meeting the patient's need for punishment, and if the assigned tasks finally irritate him to the point of verbally attacking you, the doctor, and the hospital, the attitude has done what it was intended to do—

turned the patient's anger out upon the world rather than within himself. However, should his anger suddenly flare up into a physical outburst upon you or others, it should be controlled quietly, firmly, and with *no reproach*. The doctor will then suggest further use of the attitude, which may guide the patient in more active physical release of pent-up emotions.

Is an Assumed Attitude Honest?

We have discussed a number of attitudes which we often take for granted, but when we examine them closely we may find that it will be difficult to use these attitudes with patients, who, for the most part, will be perfect strangers to us. You wonder if you can "pretend" to like a patient, not to be displeased when he spits on you, or bites you, or attempts to get your keys away. The answer is that you do not pretend an attitude; you merely utilize one of a store of the many attitudes you have tucked away in your memory. You do not have to "like" a patient, nor is it wise to pretend to do so; it is unrealistic, and we are attempting to make patients find reality inhabitable. All of us are disliked by someone or another, and it would be most artificial and unfair for the patient to find himself in a place where everyone "liked" him; it would be uncomfortable because it is unnatural. He would dislike some of the staff and would feel quite guilty if they all liked him. Be natural, show your like or dislike in a *civilized* way, always keeping in mind that this is your chosen field. If you are uncomfortable about such persons, it may be wise to utilize your talents in another branch of nursing or even in another field. Patients are a bit frightened of nurses who show complete calm at all times; it is a temptation to try that calm and see to what lengths one must go to break it. It is terrifying to find that the calm cannot be broken, because it seems unreal and inhuman. A patient once told the writer, many years ago, that she was nothing but a stuffed uniform. The nurse who attempts so to control her emotions that patients never share a human feeling with her is indeed a stuffed uniform and not a nurse.

With knowledge of how patients may feel and act, we can utilize the attitudes we have learned, or become more aware of those attitudes we always have, and give them to patients much as we give medication. The depressed, self-deprecatory patient who complains of unworthiness and guilt is in need of having that guilt mitigated, and it has been found that a firm approach, kindly dealt, will do much to help him recover. Certainly our firmness is assumed, because essentially we like most of the people with whom we work, and when the patient is an older person, worn with worries and fears, we want to help him. The kind firmness is prescribed so he may find an outlet for his hostility while discussing the reasons for that feeling with his physician, and he will recover much more rapidly if all persons working with him assume the same attitude. Assuming this attitude is the same as giving medication every three or four hours; when we give medication, all personnel who administer it give the same dosage at the required times. This will prove difficult at first until we can accept and understand that treatment is often emotional and requires more than giving pills, rubbing backs, or applying ointments.

It is hard to know which is the most difficult attitude to assume—firmness or love unsolicited. It depends largely on the individual. Some people work much better with depressed persons because they have a normal attitude of rigid firmness, based on kindliness, while others have a cheerful, easy liking for people which makes it easier for them to give the sort of attention meant by love unsolicited. Patients who are out of contact with reality try the patience of the more rigid person, and depressed patients are upsetting to the easygoing, friendly person. If you find it difficult to assume an attitude toward a particular patient or type of patient, mention this to the doctor and the charge nurse. In most hospitals they will see to it that your assignment is with the type of patient with whom you are most comfortable, as this means getting the most from you as well as your getting the most satisfaction from your work. It is more important that we be honest with ourselves and know our own emotions and feelings than to worry about the honesty of assuming an attitude.

SUGGESTED REFERENCES

Guide to the Order Sheet (mimeographed pamphlet), The Menninger Foundation, Topeka, Kans., 1946, pp. 8-17.

Render, Helena W., *Nurse-Patient Relationships in Psychiatry*, McGraw-Hill Book Company, Inc., New York, 1947, pp. 88-124.

Strecker, Edward; Ebaugh, Franklin; and Ewalt, Jack, *Practical Clinical Psychiatry*, 7th ed., The Blakiston Company, Philadelphia, 1947, pp. 451-456.

Warren, Howard C., *Dictionary of Psychology*, Houghton Mifflin Company, Boston, 1934.

CHAPTER 6

Specific Attitudes

CERTAIN ATTITUDES are good therapy for particular types of mental illness, but these same attitudes may be harmful in other situations. It is important, therefore, that we consider the use of attitudes with various kinds of patients.

The Schizophrenic Patient

Schizophrenic patients are frightened people. They are frightened of reality, of emotions, and of giving. They want to be liked, to be like other persons, and to be a part of the group, but they are so unsure of themselves that they make blunders, and they are most conscious of themselves and of those blunders. They are fearful of being laughed at, so they retreat into a world of fantasy, wherein they are the center of attention, always appear attractive, say and do just the right things to gain approval, and are never without the love they want so greatly. They are probably the loneliest people in the world.

One of the greatest mistakes in judgment any one of the professional staff can make is to believe that schizophrenic patients are happy. We hear them laughing, chuckling, or singing to themselves, watch them smear feces, dress giddily, or undress with no apparent embarrassment, scold the personnel, tell officials to go to hell, and swear, spit, and attack others as though they get great pleasure from this. Actually, they don't. Much of the singing, talking to themselves, and chuckling is an attempt to fill up the terrible void of aloneness and

SPECIFIC ATTITUDES

the feeling of being unwanted and unloved. Even when these reactions are responses to hallucinations, they are an attempt to fill this unhappy space in their lives. Their undressing, vulgarity, and decorative actions are often the acts of very small children who have not yet learned the mores of the social group in which they live.

This retreat to childlike or infantile actions is our clue to the really great unhappiness they carry with them. As children, all of us, even if we were not wanted or loved, were given a certain amount of attention, our needs were met, and we had no serious worries or problems about behaving to meet the standards of society. The schizophrenic patient, in his search for some way of life in which he may find happiness, retreats to a more childish level. In the hospital, and in the home, too, he is fed (often spoon-fed or tube-fed), taken to the toilet, washed and dressed, and watched rather closely to prevent self-injury. These are forms of attention—often the only forms he can find acceptable because he thus gains much and gives nothing.

Such a method of living is only half living, merely keeping the body alive while the mind wanders off in the wistful pastures of fantasy. We must make reality pleasant enough for the schizophrenic patient to want to remain within its realms, to be willing to give up his constant daydreaming for the everyday routines of the hospital, and gradually to build up his interest in reality to the point of being able to live in our society, using his fantasies only within normal range (release of aggression, simple wish fulfillment, etc.). To do this, we must start with the basic attitude of love unsolicited. That is, we must accept the patient as he is, an individual with a certain personality pattern which makes him different from all other individuals. Along with our acceptance, we must have a fairly thorough knowledge of his personal background, his home life, how he grew, and how he reacted to the situations which arose in his life. Acceptance, knowledge, and understanding then become the base for love unsolicited. We must know how the individual reacted to family situations, to a new sibling, to a stepparent, to a divorce, to going to school, to entering business, to getting married, or to having a baby. With such knowledge we can prevent counterparts of such situations from arising within the hospital, or, if they arise, we can know how to meet them.

We give the schizophrenic patient attention, see to his physical wants, and are ready to meet his emotional needs when we know he can accept us. There are no hard-and-fast rules for this, and many of the best doctors, nurses, and social workers have difficulty explaining their great success with schizophrenic patients. It is a "feeling," and when one has that feeling he knows it; if he hasn't the feeling, he can't get it. Not everyone can get along with schizophrenic patients, and if you are one of those persons who cannot, don't break your heart and spirit trying; work with those patients with whom you can work successfully. Perhaps the real explanation of this "feeling" is the willingness to give and give and give without expecting a return and without blaming the patient for his behavior, an ability to empathize completely with the great fear of rejection the schizophrenic always has within him. This means being ready constantly to show an interest in what the patient is doing and in his attempts to meet you. Sometimes it may mean no more than just being there, ready to greet him with a smile when he approaches, or to comment pleasantly on the weather.

Often the patient will show no response, or a response so small as to be almost imperceptible. It is a flashing shadow of a response, and again we can explain this only by saying it is a feeling, a sort of awareness that for a second, or a moment, the patient was with you, unafraid and pleased. This may be followed by days of apparent unresponsiveness, but we must never show regret or annoyance that he seems withdrawn again. For the patient to make even so small an effort at responding to another human being is a step forward. He is like the sea anemone which puts out frail tendrils in the ocean but withdraws them when the slightest shadow passes over the water. Our job is to keep from frightening him, so the ten-

SPECIFIC ATTITUDES

drils will remain out, soaking up the approval and warmth of our being there, gaining strength in this contact, and losing fear of further contacts.

I recall a mute patient who sat quietly in her room day after day, finally responding to the repeated invitation to come and sit by the desk. For hours the patient would sit there, apparently staring into nothingness, saying nothing, doing nothing; then she would rise and return to her room. I would thank her for the visit and tell her to return again. This went on for weeks, occasionally with my saying something about the weather, the view from the window, or just what a nice meal lunch had been. One day the patient responded with a smile, and in a couple of days she talked shyly about paintings she had seen in Paris. Her embroidery became the subject of long discussions about coloring, and what threads to use, and how it would look, and once she grinned wryly and said she had been working on that piece for ten years. She never did make any further stitches on it, but the opening human contact had been made, and other members of the nursing and adjunctive personnel were gradually accepted by her. Today, some years later, this patient still remains in the hospital, but she has improved to the point of going into town for dinner or a show, to taking an occasional trip with a companion, to playing a fair game of tennis, and to joining groups of patients in such social activities as parties and teas. She is not cured, of course, but here is a patient who is no longer so frightened that she remains totally alone, unable to make any contacts with reality. Though she is still fearful of reality, she is living more comfortably among the many people with whom she must come in contact.

Perhaps some patients cannot be returned to society, but our care of the ill is not aimed exclusively to that end. We must face the fact that many patients with all sorts of illnesses are unable to return to the "normal" world outside. We must also face the task of making these persons as comfortable and happy as possible, as sure of the rights of human dignity within the hospital's walls as the so-called "normal" person is without. The schizophrenic must be surrounded with love, warmth, and a feeling of worth as a human being. With this feeling as a base for further treatment, much of his being "cured" will then depend upon his ability as a person to make the adjustment of standing alone and accepting people outside the hospital.

This latter part of treatment is now being called rehabilitation or resocialization. It has been found that many patients who were heretofore kept within the confines of the hospital can make an adjustment which allows them to live outside and work or attend school, returning to the hospital only for guidance or help, or perhaps having to return to the hospital at night to sleep. There is a great deal to be done in this endeavor; we are only beginning to try day hospital plans, and to enlarge our mental-health clinics so that many of these schizophrenic persons need never enter the hospital for full-time care. This is good, because it is very easy for the schizophrenic person to become so dependent upon hospitals that he will not make any effort to leave.

This leads to the problem of deciding when we must be realistic with such patients, and how much asocial behavior we can accept without showing displeasure or disapproval. No matter how sick the person, or how frightened, we must make our attitudes fit within the situation. We must not make it appear that asocial behavior is totally acceptable. The best approach is to make socially acceptable behavior worth while by simple rewards, which vary with the individual and may be simply a pleasant smile or indulgently overlooking some infraction of a rule. The reward may be a longer visit with the patient when he is acceptable, reading some favorite book, making an effort to find a favorite record for his pleasure, or taking him for a walk about the grounds. To show displeasure without frightening him, such small things may be withheld, or he may be told he had better remain in his room until he can get along better with the group. This is not punitive, and it gives him opportunity for thought as to how his reactions turn upon himself.

SPECIFIC ATTITUDES

Again, how each situation is met will depend on the patient, his doctor's orders, and the nurse's ability to interpret the orders. The nurse must have a full understanding of what the doctor means when certain attitudes are specified. These patients need warmth and friendliness and endless patience, and under all the attitudes you will use with the schizophrenic, love must exist, just as the mother loves the child whom she may have to punish for some misdeed. The nurse must know when the patient's actions are so much a part of his illness that he cannot understand his treatment, and when his actions are a testing of her liking for him. She must, above all, be *consistent* in her treatment of him, remaining friendly even when it is necessary to isolate him from the group or to put him in some form of restraint.

The disturbed patient who must be kept in his room should not be made to feel neglected or punished. Frequent attention can be given by taking care of his wants, asking if he'd like to go to the bathroom or if he would like a glass of milk, a cookie, or some other simple treat. Suggesting that he might enjoy a magazine while he is alone, and even reading to him, are forms of showing that the nurse likes him and is trying to help while he is going through a rather difficult time of getting along with people. All too often the isolated patient is left totally alone, and his feeling of being rejected is pretty well founded.

The busy nurse must recognize her own feelings and face the fact that the relief she feels when disturbed patients are isolated is not exactly good nursing care. It is too easy to assume that the patient who is doing no mischief is "good," when actually it may be a most fearful and tragic experience for him, and he may need the companionship of others. That companionship is best given by the personnel, who understand his illness and who can give a measured and controlled amount of attention without exciting him to further disturbance.

Even the schizophrenic patient who is destructive and hostile will respond to a consistently helpful approach. He may take great delight in ripping rags, which may be used later to make braided rugs. He can release much of his hostility while tearing the rags, and it helps him to know that they can be put to a useful purpose later. The same rags can be kept and utilized in his treatment by getting him to dye them at a time when he is able to work with such material. He will probably recognize that these are the things he tore up while he was so disturbed, and may even joke about it or, more important, may start to talk about why he tore them and why he was disturbed at that time. The alert nurse or occupational therapist can note these conversations, which may prove useful to the doctor in treatment or in preventing further hostile outbursts.

Every action and remark of the schizophrenic patient is a symptom of his problems, and, although there is universal sameness in the basic pattern of schizophrenia, the individual patient has his own responses and personal pattern which are entirely different from the next person's. The psychiatric nurse must recognize this fact, and this recognition will keep her from allowing such a patient to remain in isolation unattended except for meals and trips to the toilet. That would be analogous to pulling the covers over a patient whose incision is seeping blood. It makes the bed look tidy but leads to dangerous consequences.

The Depressed Patient

The depressed and suicidal patient is also a frightened person, but his method of meeting fears is quite different from withdrawing into a fantasy world to find love. He rejects love, saying he is not worthy of it, and he expresses guilt when any act of love is proffered. He often has strong guilt feelings about his inability to meet the demands and high standards of maturity, and instead of blaming the world for these feelings, he turns the blame inward upon himself. He becomes self-punitive and spends much time thinking of or expressing his unworthiness: "If it were not for me, my wife and family would be happy"; "If I hadn't married against my family's

SPECIFIC ATTITUDES

desires, they would be happy"; "If I could only be the businessman my boss seems to think I am by giving me this responsible job, things would be much better." Such thoughts become more intense and self-punitive, until the person says, "If I were dead, everybody would be much better off, including me." They may be expressed by mute withdrawal into a negative state, such as refusing to eat, bathe, or converse, or the state may be negative but not mute, and the patient will say he cannot eat because he is unworthy. He may keep away from others because he is "not clean," or he may complain of having a bad odor, or of lacking certain internal organs (often the throat, stomach, or intestines). He may go even further and attempt suicide.

The desire for suicide is complicated by mixed unconscious feelings. The person who attempts to kill himself does two things: he removes his "unworthy" person from the world, thereby punishing the world for not understanding him and his needs, and he punishes himself for being such a hostile person. As children, most of us have thought of dying with a mixture of pain and pleasure. When we were scolded for some misdeed, we thought, "I'll just die, and they'll be sorry," and often the thought was accompanied by a great deal of fantasy of the family's sorrow, and our own tragic and innocent little body laid out in great pomp. This is so typical that writers use it frequently for moving or amusing scenes in their works. One of the best descriptions of the reaction is in Mark Twain's wonderful section of *Tom Sawyer*, where Tom and his friend Huck have been missing for days, and funeral services are being held in the church. The two boys have returned to town, and creep into the choir loft to hear their own services. They are so touched by them that they sob aloud and are, of course, discovered. The sorrow of the townspeople turns to irritation. It is a remarkably clear picture of the mechanisms of depression and guilt reactions.

Recognition of deep-seated guilt feelings helps the nurse to meet the patient's needs in the most therapeutic manner, one of which is to avoid back-patting and comforting the depressed person. When he is declaiming his guilt and unworthiness, it does no good whatsoever to reassure him that he is not unworthy of attention. This only makes him feel more guilty and unworthy. A fairly rigid program of work and expected compliance to hospital routine should be set up, and we use the attitude of kind firmness in planning the routine.

Accompanying this attitude, the doctor may order a full schedule of helpful and menial tasks, *to which we must make the patient adhere.* At first, he may go quietly on with the tasks—which range from emptying ash trays and wastebaskets to the dull routines of making dressings or mopping the floors —but soon an interesting change will take place. He will begin to complain about the tasks, about our cruelty in making him carry out such unpleasant jobs, and about the cruelty and lack of understanding in us, his family, and the world in general. This complaining is healthy. At last, the patient is turning his irritation outward. Heretofore, he had these feelings about events in his life situation, but he had kept them to himself, blaming himself for the many small disturbances in his routines, and that self-blame led to guilt and feelings of unworthiness. It is at this point that we must *not* make any change in the routine. Let the patient gripe, and, if possible, agree with him that the tasks are dirty, monotonous, and even trivial, but necessary, and *keep him at them.* Often, patients recognize the value of such tasks and, when feeling particularly unhapy, will ask for an especially nasty job.

I know of several occasions when patients learned the helpfulness of hard, menial work. One very depressed young man kept to himself, quoted terrifying, punitive chapters from the Bible, and wrung his hands in great agitation, tears running down his cheeks. We assigned him to scrubbing the back steps of the ward, under supervision *always*, and made no comment about his agitation. Sometimes he scrubbed those steps three times a day. He began to improve, and we were amused and touched when he would suddenly leave the

SPECIFIC ATTITUDES

group, where he had begun to join in the conversation, come to the nursing office, and request the scrubbing brush and bucket. He improved to the point of being discharged to his family, and assured us he would meet any further depression by hard work. "It really helps," he said.

Many women do this sort of thing without being told it is therapeutic. How often do we hear women say, "I felt so blue today, I washed all the woodwork in the house"? Often, when we are faced with a special task we don't like to carry out, we get into quite a little whirlwind of other activities, and the mending that has been waiting for weeks, the polishing of silver, the cleaning of bureau drawers, which we had been putting off, get done rapidly. Once over, the special task seems less impossible to carry out. All that we in psychiatry have done is utilize this factor in treating the depressed patient. The person who has become so depressed that he is a danger to himself is beyond the point of being able to plan such activity, and we must plan it for him. This "need for punishment" can advance to a degree wherein the patient will refuse food and have to be tube-fed, a most unpleasant procedure. He may attempt to show his need for punishment in such a way that he will force us into the position of bodily carrying him to his activities, to bathing him, and to acting so firmly that he will feel he is being punished. It is important that we carry out such activities kindly. That is why we speak of *kind* firmness.

One of the most important things to remember about working with depressed patients is that they will improve, in spite of themselves, under such a regime, and *with improvement, they reach the most dangerous peak of illness*. While they are so terribly depressed and agitated, we watch them constantly, but as soon as they begin to show signs of more "normal" behavior, to laugh once in a while, to hold normal conversations without reference to self-guilt, we think they are better. Before, they were too engrossed in self-pity and condemnation to do much about it, often retreating to a mute and negativistic level. Now, they are expressing hostility more freely, the guilt is free-floating, *and the danger of suicide is at its greatest*. Constant watchfulness must be continued if we are to prevent tragedy. This is so difficult to explain to persons new to the field of psychiatry, to the family, indeed to the patient, that it takes all the skill the psychiatrist and social worker have to prevent families from taking the patient home when he reaches this point. All too often, if the patient is taken home against advice, or the personnel let up on their watchfulness, a suicide results. The comment the family and personnel almost invariably make is: "He seemed so much better." We cannot stress strongly enough that when the depressed patient begins to improve, it is imperative to watch him more closely than ever.

Kind firmness is a helpful attitude to know for many situations other than the active nursing care of depressed patients. You will notice that patients often ask for the nurse who has been most firm (in a pleasant way) to them, that people will turn for help to the friend who is consistently firm. Children respond well to such persons, too, for pleasant firmness *consistently* shown gives them a feeling of security. Everyone likes to feel that the person in immediate charge of his care offers security, even if he may rebel against it at times.

The depressed patient may become extremely agitated and restless, and at these times he is of great danger to himself. His erratic activity lends itself well to suicidal attempts, often bizarre but most real. The firmness and the rigid routine implied by kind firmness are most helpful to such persons—an anchor for their seemingly purposeless activities. The patient who goes from withdrawn depression into overactivity is usually fighting off tremendous guilt feelings and self-destructive ideas. It is as if he feels he will not be able to consider suicide if he keeps active. He may chatter constantly, or pick at himself, at his clothing, or at the furniture.

One patient who had periodic attacks of such restlessness spent hours of her day taking the drawers out of her bureau and piling them up on the floor, scattering her clothes about,

SPECIFIC ATTITUDES

and talking incessantly. She was obsessed with a desire to disrobe herself, and felt extremely guilty about it, and the piling of bureau drawers and scattering of their contents was a defense against disrobing. When she began to tear up her clothing and increased in agitation until it was necessary to remove all furniture from her room, her doctor told her she might undress if she wished, that we would understand. This satisfied her, and she remained in her room, totally nude, singing quietly to herself. Picking at her skin was met by giving her some old clothing to tear into rags, which were later dyed and woven into a rug. Since her behavior was most asocial, she was kept in her room, but the nurse went in to visit her frequently, sitting on the floor and talking quietly. A favorite poem, Joyce Kilmer's *Trees,* had a soothing effect upon her, and the nurse recited it over and over again. Long after the period of agitation was past, the patient commented on the nurse's willingness to spend so much time with her "when I was naughty" and added how helpful the poem had been. She added, "You were always so kind." Those few simple words were ample reward for the hours and hours of reciting the poem, of sitting on the floor and sharing the patient's meal hour, of firmly refusing to allow her to run about the corridor nude, or to interfere with other patients.

The nurse must remember that kind firmness is not rigid control of all the patient's activity. The agitation is an expression of great internal conflict, and the pressure is so great that it must be released. Restraint of such an agitated patient may hold him in check physically (though a great deal of harm can be done to such patients by use of restraint), but it does nothing to help resolve the emotional furor causing the activity. When restraint is necessary, it should be used matter-of-factly and for the patient's security, *not for the feeling of security it gives the nurse.* Working with the mentally ill is rarely conducive to a feeling of great security. The unexpected is a constant occurrence. The nurse must feel a great enough inner sureness about the treatment and have such a genuine love for people that she can rely upon her knowledge of the individual patient rather than upon mechanical restraint.

Anxiety and Fear

The nurse in the general hospital will see more anxiety and fear than depression, and there is a great difference, but both are equally important to recognize, and firm kindness is helpful in meeting either. While depression is considered truly morbid, or a symptom of severe illness, anxiety and fear are considered "normal," in that everyone has periods of one or the other, and they are related usually to expected events which arouse uncertainty and apprehension. Both anxiety and fear will give rise to certain physiological reactions with which the nurse is familiar. The sympathetic nervous system reacts to these two emotions by giving any one or a combination of symptoms: trembling, sweating, dilated pupils, nausea, hiccuping, cold extremities, or rapid pulse. The patient may not express himself verbally at all.

An observant nurse will notice these symptoms and tactfully lead to a discussion of the patient's hospital care, which, in turn, may cause him to reveal his fears. Such simple questions as "Have you ever been in a hospital before?" or "Have you ever used a bedpan?" can relieve the tension. The patient's answer will lead to further, seemingly idle chitchat, and, like most of us, he will feel better for the conversation.

Treatments and tests, which we tend to discuss glibly, may be most frightening to the patient, and the nurse should always ask the patient if he knows what is meant by the long names he has had thrown at him. So simple a test as a B. M. R. means nothing to a lay person, and the fact that he is told not to smoke, drink any fluid, or move more than necessary after midnight can rouse all sorts of fantastic notions, which will affect the basal metabolic rate more than if he were physically active. A calm, simple explanation will put him at ease and assure a more accurate testing.

This is true of practically all the tests and treatments with which we are familiar. We must remember that the patient is a guest in our hospital, and extending ordinary courtesy to him will allay many fears and anxieties. Insofar as possible, his requests to see members of his family, the clergy, or the doctor should be granted. If such requests seem overweighted with emotion (querulousness, irritability, or dread), try talking with him about the requests. Discussion is always a good treatment for ordinary anxieties and fears, but patients may be afraid to talk about their feelings lest we may be amused. No fear, no matter how farfetched we may think it, is amusing. Patients entering hospitals have all sorts of fantasies of mutilation and death which we too may have had, but we exchanged these ideas for our working knowledge of hospitals. If we *empathize* with the patient, put ourselves in his place by really *feeling* his emotions, we can understand how distressed he is, and, as always, understanding and knowledge are our tools to aid people to recover.

The Psychoneurotic Patient

Psychoneurotic patients are often the most difficult to care for because we tend to think the patient is just pretending his illness. While it is true that his physical complaints may have no organic basis, or that they may be very small compared to the degree of incapacity he has, we must remember that his emotional problems are so great that they cause his complaints, and the *organic complaint must be taken into consideration*. It is often through caring for his physical illness that we get the first opportunity to approach his emotional problems. One basic fact about the diagnosis of psychoneurosis is that the patient's problems are of such a frightening aspect that he has had to develop a physical complaint to keep himself from recognizing his emotional difficulties. Not all nurses can work well with such patients, and if you find that they make you irritable or caustic in comment, it is wise to switch to the care of a different type of patient.

Psychoneurotic patients need understanding too, of course, and kindliness, but often the kindliness must be meted out much differently from the way we give it to the schizophrenic.

We must learn how to ignore physical complaints without being insulting or derogatory; we must give physical care without making it the alpha and omega of the patient's hospitalization; and we must learn to listen endlessly to physical complaints without falling into the temptation of telling our own physical problems, or discussing other patients we have known who had similar and worse ailments. Matter-of-factness is useful here, and a cheerful "the world won't end" attitude is effective when the patient complains of his sore throat, his constipation, or his nervous stomach.

Sometimes the doctor will ask us to be indulgent until the patient learns we are not going to strip his physical illness from him in one swift gesture. It is wise to recognize that many people make a social adjustment if they have some physical complaint to fall back on when society's pressure is too great for them to meet. That headache we develop when we don't want to attend some function, the upset stomach, the irritability accompanying some task we either openly dislike or unconsciously wish not to do—all these are nothing more nor less than the same sort of physical complaint the psychoneurotic patient has. We know how we like to be treated at such times, and the simplest attitude to adopt for the care of psychoneurotic patients is one we would like to have applied to us if we were in the patient's place. We should be sympathetic, helpful, and noncondemning, and we should not discuss the complaints at any great length. True, it is easier to be sympathetic and nonjudgmental to the friend who has an occasional headache when faced with something unpleasant than it is to the hospitalized patient whose complaints are fairly constant, and who demands much attention.

The psychoneurotic patient who is in the hospital is a person whose physical complaints have so disabled him that he is no longer able to compete in reality, or he is a person who recognizes, or has had recognition brought to him, that much of his trouble is emotional. He is in great need of passive friendliness and of support and encouragement in his simplest endeavors. Since the psychiatrist often will be

SPECIFIC ATTITUDES 63

making an effort to refocus the patient's energy away from his physical complaints, we should not be solicitous or giving of unsolicited love. Here, we must wait patiently, be ready should the patient need our attention, and then give it in a friendly but not too concerned manner. By eliminating the physical ailment as the center of attention, by not allowing the patient to use this as his only means of getting attention, and by treating it as a sort of everyday and to-be-expected occurrence, we remove his central unrealistic theme of attention-getting, at the same time that the doctor is helping him to discover and accept the emotional conflicts which led him to utilize bodily ailments as escape mechanisms.

Such patients tend to be irritable, to arouse hostility in those around them, or to be whining and complaintive. Only the mature, stable nurse with a good sense of humor and genuine warmth can work well with these people. Sternness frightens such patients, as they feel they are being unjustifiably punished, and they will retreat into their complaints or become pettily nagging.

Psychoneurotic patients react very well to routines and will often be sticklers for receiving medication exactly on time, will question the contents of medication bottles, will be querulous about their food and toilet habits, fussy about their appearance and the appearance of their rooms, and, all in all, pretty trying persons to work with day after day. Here, if the nurse can make her friendliness impersonal, the patients respond well. They are too self-engrossed to make friendships as deeply involved as the schizophrenic patient, and they are often the patients who will have favorite nurses and doctors, make many requests, give little gifts to their "favorite" staff members, promise to keep in touch with them, and even do so after leaving the hospital, then promptly drop all correspondence within a very brief period. Their habit of playing favorites is a dangerous one, and the nurse must be careful to avoid this by not allowing herself to be so flattered at being liked by a crotchety patient that she plays this up. Self-effacement is always difficult, especially so when an irritable patient tells you no one else ever rubbed his back better, or made him feel more comfortable, or "saved his life." (This is an expression many psychoneurotic patients use freely and is a guide to how seriously minor mishaps affect them.) We have a tendency to try to encourage this by making greater and greater efforts to please that individual. Perhaps only experience can stop us from making this mistake, but, as much as possible, try to treat all such patients with no more and no less attention than you give to others.

Nursing these patients can be most rewarding because they often have great ingenuity and wit when they have overcome their absorption with their physical ailments, and they frequently have interests which can be utilized by the nurse to draw them away from discussion of physical ills. They are people who are much aware of reality, rather than greatly withdrawn from it, and one treatment problem is their tendency to intellectualize. Here is a trap the nurse must beware especially. They will often start a vague, general discussion about the body or some illness, based on a magazine or newspaper article. If she watches this, the nurse can see that such discussion is leading to the patient's own problem, or that he is gleaning new facts to utilize later when he is faced with emotional difficulties he wishes to avoid. It is wise to change the subject as gracefully as possible when such discussions arise, and you may suggest he take it up with the doctor. Group discussions of ailments among psychoneurotic patients should also be discouraged as tactfully as possible. Tact, good-natured firmness, and humor are quite a big combination, but they are most useful in nursing all patients, and especially those who are psychoneurotic.

The Feeble-minded Patient

Although many states separate the feeble-minded from psychiatric patients, one frequently finds them in the psychiatric unit for diagnosis, in the infirmary because of some minor physical ailment, or even in the general hospital for treatment of physical illness. They present special problems, largely because they have the minds of children in the bodies of adults. We are prone to take persons at their surface value, forgetting that these patients are literally unable to meet the standards of adult life, not because of emotional difficulties but because they simply do not have the brain power to go beyond the very simple basic ability to keep alive. This basic ability is to eat, sleep, and respond to normal affection. Beyond this, serious problems may develop. Since the adult body makes certain sexual demands (which in the normal adult can either be sublimated, or met in full awareness of what is involved), the feeble-minded present a social problem. They may become involved with the sexually aberrant or may have children whom they are not properly equipped to rear.

This problem is being met in some states with sterilization of the feeble-minded—a solution which is not always considered morally and legally sound. Whether or not feeble-mindedness is inherited is still being questioned, and it is not my purpose to take a stand on this issue. It seems more important to recognize that such persons are unable to meet the diverse and complicated demands of rearing children in our present society, and it is most unfair to such children. Marked emotional problems arise which then become the problems of the society in which these families live. Therefore, how to treat the feeble-minded is an important problem of which all citizens should be aware. What steps the state or civic government may take are important to all of us, and, as good citizens, we must give some thought to the matter.

Recognition that the feeble-minded are incapable of handling adult affairs is important, but mere recognition of the fact and attempts to isolate them do not solve the problem entirely. It was found in England, during World War II, that many of these persons could do useful work in the labor field, provided the job was not too complicated and good supervision was given them. This has opened new possibilities in the care and treatment of the feeble-minded. Recent experiments in psychiatry have attempted to educate the class of feeble-minded ranking below the moron group, and some studies in hormonal therapy have been carried out. To date, we know that many of the persons we thought were unteachable can be taught the simple principles of self-care; that under supervision they can play in groups, keep themselves from becoming soiled, and lead very restricted but rather happy lives. Often these persons must be institutionalized, and it is with the care of institutionalized feeble-minded persons that these paragraphs are mostly concerned.

Patience and understanding are again the basic principles of good care. We must know just how limited these persons are, how incapable of keeping up with our very rigid standards of societal living and ordinary give and take. Like children, they have little conception of time; abstract thinking of the simplest sort is pretty much beyond their grasp; and a fairly rigid pattern of life, kept to its simplest, will help greatly in group control of these patients. It is important to remember that a rigid pattern of group life *does not eliminate affection*. In fact, such rigidity means that the nurses or attendants should give more affection. If toilet training and meal schedules are rigidly adhered to, it means that the patients require less reprimanding for soiling, eat well, and get to know by physical signs that it is time for certain bodily functions. Such a pattern allows the nurse or attendant to plan the "in-between times" so that these patients are content and happy, and are doing such constructive work as they are able to handle. There may be classroom instruction for those capable of benefiting by it; there may be instruction or supervision in simple farm work or work in the institution's laundry or kitchen. Such work should be remunerated as the local situation permits, but it is always within the province of any supervisor to give praise as well as pay, and these patients need praise and approval for the simplest of accomplishments. Breaking the patterns of toilet training, or eating, or group living, should be met with disapproval, kindly given; but punishment should be eliminated from the program unless it is the withholding of some privilege for a short period. Like very small children, if punished, feeble-minded persons should be punished immediately so they know what it is for, and once punished, the matter should be dropped.

Conversation, games, and training for personal hygiene should be kept at a simple level, with not too much competition. Temper tantrums are not unusual with these persons, and it is best to meet them firmly, kindly, and by isolation. It is wise to remember at this time that to withhold a treat or favorite dessert would only be baffling to the patient. The tantrum must be met immediately, and disapproval should be shown at that moment, for the memory span of the feebleminded is not very great, and the withheld dessert, or some other form of reprisal for the tantrum, if given at a later time, will only lead to his thinking he is being picked on, and for no known reason. It is most wise, too, to remember that these persons with the minds of small children have the bodies of adults and can become dangerous to themselves or others if tantrums are unchecked. As they become used to institutionalization, and as they are met with kindliness and friendliness, they may be less apt to have any aggressive outbursts, but since they do quarrel among themselves, constant supervision must be maintained. In their work, they must never use dangerous equipment—no matches (though they may smoke), knives, or similar tools—and it almost goes without saying that they should not be allowed to operate complicated machinery or equipment which may endanger them or others should unexpected situations arise. Plan work which they are capable of handling, praise them liberally, give much attention, keep a routine, and be endlessly patient; the results will be amazing in the socialization of the feeble-minded, *within their individual mental limits.*

Organic Brain Damage

Neurologists and psychiatrists still tend to discuss rather heatedly whether the patient with organic brain damage belongs in the psychiatric hospital or in the general hospital. As less and less stigma is attached to mental illness, society will be better able to accept the fact that the patient with extensive organic damage to his brain may be legally "insane" (dependent on the extent and location of the damage); that is, that he is incapable of using good judgment in carrying out his personal and business affairs. It stands to reason that a person who loses a limb is less able to carry out the work he formerly did with all his limbs, though he may be greatly aided by prostheses. Similarly, a person who loses a portion of his brain through disease or injury is less able to carry out the normal function of his body which is controlled by that part of his brain. No method has been found to replace brain tissue, and we know that certain areas of the brain control emotions, judgment, and memory recall, all of which are most important in our daily living. Persons with brain damage may be so seriously affected that they may need a guardian appointed for them, or they may show little more than slight memory lapses. The type of behavior pattern shown by such patients depends on the location of the damage, the extent of damage, and the *personality pattern* of the individual. He must be treated physically, of course, and symptomatically for the behavior problem he presents.

Behavior Problems

Persons with asocial behavior are difficult to handle anywhere, and in the hospital they become a problem because they may incite psychotic patients to destructive behavior or help them to gain access to weapons, alcohol, or release. The patient presenting behavior problems usually is not psychotic, and, because of this, the staff may find it hard to understand and accept his actions.

Alcoholism. The alcoholic patient is only one of the types of serious behavior disorders with which the staff has to cope. With him, our patience often gives out because he will be a model of good behavior for long periods of time and then break down. During his period of good behavior he is often a gregarious, charming person, and may help with ward work, assist other patients, and in general "get in good" with the staff. In fact, it is such action that nurses and aides

SPECIFIC ATTITUDES

must guard against accepting too wholeheartedly, for the patient will use his good behavior and his contribution to peace and quiet on the ward as an excuse for being released from the minor irritants of ward routines such as not having matches, going to bed at the regular bedtime, etc. Many persons seem unable to grasp the fact that the alcoholic is not addicted to alcohol on a conscious level, that he doesn't just turn to drink and then get too much and misbehave. Deep unconscious motives are present which make him seek alcohol as surely as the schizophrenic seeks happiness in his fantasy world, and these motives must be understood before the disturbing symptoms and acting out can be understood.

We have learned that schizophrenics are unhappy and frightened and turn to their fantasies as a method of getting some satisfaction. The alcoholic, too, is frightened and unhappy, but he attempts to bolster his self-confidence and tries to gain status in society by resorting to alcohol. He often feels he can "be himself" with a couple of drinks in him, often because the depressant action of the alcohol dulls his sensitivity and he becomes less aware of the many realities which frighten him. He voices his opinion of his boss, his wife, or other relatives, and the dulled nervous system does not nag him with guilt at the time.

After such a bout with alcohol he is very apt to be extremely guilty and depressed and often quite suicidal. The hostile feelings were there all the time, and his lack of awareness of them under the influence of alcohol did not eliminate them. As the nerves recover from the dulled state, the hostility and accompanying guilt flood him with a fresh impact, and he has a tendency to want to return to the drink which keeps him from this awareness. He is actually a child who has never grown emotionally beyond the breast or bottle stage of his life, and he seeks comfort from sucking.

These persons will "suck in" the unwary nurse or aide by appearing childlike and in need of mothering; in fact, many persons marry alcoholics with the idea that they can reform them. Nothing is further from the truth, for these patients demand so much that it is almost impossible to meet their needs. Few human beings, if any, can spend their entire lives mothering a suckling infant. Our own dependent needs, our own desires to be coddled and understood, are too great for us to give and give and give as constantly as the alcoholic patient demands. The first failure to meet his demands will result in disappointment to him, and he will return to his unfailing friend, the bottle. Then the tragic cycle of remorse, guilt, surface devil-may-care attitude, and hostility starts again. In the hospital such patients are not too difficult to control when alcohol can be kept from them, but their need frequently becomes great enough for them to attempt to bribe their way out, to try to steal the keys, to attack personnel.

Most alcoholic patients are in the hospital under the pressure of relatives or others close to them: the wife (or husband) who threatens divorce if the patient doesn't stop drinking, the family who threaten to break all ties, the business associate who threatens to break off business connections, ad infinitum. This in itself is a tremendous pressure which does nothing to lessen the burden of fear and insecurity the alcoholic person always has present.

The group called Alcoholics Anonymous has done wonderful things in aiding the alcoholic patient and in revealing to us what makes the patient act as he does. The first requisite to join AA is sincerity of purpose. The group has recognized that unless the individual himself realizes fully that he has a problem in his drinking, little can be done. This is true, too, in hospitalization, and there are not many hospitals which will admit alcoholics as long-term-treatment patients because of the many problems which arise. The voluntary admission has come because he acknowledges his need for help, and it is the opening wedge to aiding him. The entire staff must understand and co-operate with this tragic person, not condemning him when he does go out and get drunk; not punishing him by their attitudes. The alcoholic punishes himself, often sustaining injuries to his body as well as to his emotions, and while his deep guilt feelings following a bout should be

SPECIFIC ATTITUDES

met with firmness rather than commiseration, he should not be treated punitively.

Some hospitals now use the assistance of AA members in the care of alcoholic patients, and the nurse and aides should know about this organization—its basic rules, aims, and accomplishments, as well as how to reach the head of the local chapter in an emergency. Should a patient be a member of AA, in the hospital for other treatment, the doctor will let the staff know if he plans to use him in helping other patients. Sometimes it is a most useful and effective tool, and often the alcoholic patient who will not respond to treatment by doctors or psychologists will co-operate for a fellow alcoholic patient who has started his recovery through AA.

Drug Addiction. The behavior of drug addicts is somewhat like alcoholics, and the nurse and attendants must be on guard at all times against the charming manners and pleasant ways of the patient who will try to win over to his side some one member of the staff. There are several important differences which must be kept in mind. First, narcotic addicts are subject to the Federal Narcotics Act, and persons helping such people to get narcotics are playing with fire. Second, narcotic addicts are very apt to have acute withdrawal symptoms, go into convulsive states, shock, and death if they are withdrawn from a drug too rapidly. The nurse *must* follow the doctor's orders meticulously in giving drugs to such persons, no matter what her personal feelings are about people addicted to narcotics. In drug addiction, as in all other illnesses, we must know something of the basic personality pattern. Much like the alcoholic, these persons have not completely grown up and must have some artificial stimulant to keep them going. The fact that their choice of drugs is not always a stimulant does not mean much. The stimulus lies in their knowing they will get a release from their unwanted emotional turmoil by taking the drug of their choice.

These persons are often pleasant, winning, and well-mannered when feeling at all well, but on being crossed, disappointed in some minor activity, or meeting the inflexibility of certain hospital regulations, they will revert to whining, argumentative, hostile, and often combative activity. They will lie, steal, and injure to obtain the drug they need so intensely. They cannot be trusted; they know this and dislike it, and will vent their hostility on the hospital personnel. They are often the sort of persons who are right while the rest of the world is wrong, and, although friendliness is indicated, it must be a guarded sort, with rigid application of rules at all times and immediate reporting of any suspicious behavior, even if it involves another staff member. These addicts are dangerous to themselves, and certainly to others. While under the influence of drugs they will do all sorts of antisocial things including homicide, and while they are in the hospital, they are the responsibility of every member of the hospital team, from the lowest to the highest. Our guarded friendliness should be consistent, since consistency is the one thing these persons have not had in their lives. They usually have exhibited a pattern of charming likable behavior, gaining friends and love, but then, because of some frustration, have turned to drugs, and their resultant guilt and antisocial behavior have lost them these friends and their love. The consistent friendliness of the staff can lead to genuine attempts to get away from dependency on the drug, and, as with alcoholism, the basic requirement for getting well is the real desire to do so. We must give care to such persons on a nonjudgmental basis; we must listen to them and to their excuses for the need for a drug with no comment, and we must watch them closely and constantly at all times. We must be on guard against their attempts to get the drug they need; regulations concerning locked medicine cupboards and service-room doors must be rigidly adhered to. If we suspect they have obtained drugs, we must report it immediately, no matter how we think the drug was obtained.

Don Juanism. These persons are not often encountered in civilian hospitals, though occasionally a patient enters the hospital for treatment for behavior problems and shows a history of frequent marriages and divorces, or many love

SPECIFIC ATTITUDES

affairs. Such people usually have much personal charm, a reasonable amount of good looks, and a great "line." We find them in both sexes, and the personnel must be on guard against the personal charm of these persons, who dislike regulations and will attempt to get around them on the basis of friendship. Sexual promiscuity will lead these patients to attempt to seduce members of the staff. If you are unsure of yourself in the presence of this behavior, make every effort to avoid being alone with these patients and to keep your own behavior strictly on the professional side. Sexual relations with patients by any member of hospital personnel are not only professionally frowned upon but can lead to many legal complications. Don Juans are often children emotionally, looking upon sexual promiscuity as a method of proving they are "grown up," but their choice of partners, as well as their inability to make a stable marriage, shows how wrong this thinking is. Their emotional immaturity is seen in temper tantrums and disagreeable behavior when things are not going their way, as well as in occasional bouts of drinking when they are permitted out of the hospital.

Guarded friendliness is the attitude to give such persons. They need friendliness, but they must learn to earn it and to appreciate it for its own sake rather than for the purely selfish reason of getting out of their friendships what they can. We meet these patients when disgusted families have them committed to see if something can't be done for them, or when they are brought in by the police for having run afoul of the law in forgetting to get a divorce before remarrying, or for not supporting children by previous or present wives. Since they are rarely voluntary admissions, we must combat their fearfulness and hostility with friendliness and a matter-of-fact presentation of rules and regulations. We *must* be consistent in our approach to them and *nonjudgmental,* despite our personal convictions about their affairs.

Lying. This is a most difficult problem in the psychiatric hospital and one which can cause a great deal of trouble to all staff members. Basically, we must know why the individual patient is lying, and we must remain nonjudgmental about it. Usually it is a symptom of his maladjustment and must be treated like one, regardless of our personal feelings or even of our being involved in the lie. We must also understand why people lie. They usually do it to gain attention or to bolster their own inadequate feelings. Some lies are protective so the person telling them won't feel that he has blundered or been stupid, and these lies are not recognized as such by the person telling them. When serious consequences are the result of a lie, it is necessary to point these out, quietly and without loss of temper, and to explain that the truth will clear matters and make it easier to solve the problem which caused the original lie.

As professional persons, our initial job is to so arrange ward routines, management, and the handling of such things as keys, medicines, and special permits that the patient will not be forced by our inadequacies into a position of lying. Therefore, we must know whether certain medications have been given, certain passes permitted, what we have done with the keys, and where all members of the personnel and patients are at all times. Our written and verbal reports must be complete and accurate, even if they appear to show negligence on the part of any staff member, for with these reports the doctor can do much to determine if the patient is lying, and if so, why.

A patient's lies will range from the simple and rather childish statement that he has bathed this day to accusations of mistreatment by personnel. Each lie must be acted upon separately, depending upon the real meaning and importance of it. The little "white" lie by the patient who doesn't want to bathe today often can be overlooked with no comment. Calmness and nonpunitive attitudes are of great importance in handling lying, and measures must be taken under the advice of the physician to prevent repetition of lies or serious involvements. The nurse should not repeat or recall lies to a patient when she suspects him of being involved in further similar activities. Many of them forget yesterday's actions, and to be reminded of them is bewildering, or frightening, or humiliating. Since lies are often apt to lead to annoyances, both petty and great, we tend to show temper. Some patients will rely on this to keep up their attention-getting or to stir up excitement in an otherwise dull hospital world. The normal routines should not be so rigid that a patient is forced to lie to escape an impossible situation, and questions regarding routines, medications, or treatments should be so worded by the nurse that the patient is not tempted or pushed into lying. Working with patients who resort to lies takes endless patience, calmness, and good humor.

The lies of the schizophrenic patient are rather like the tall tales of children and can be met cheerfully and jocularly unless they become involved in paranoid detail. At this point it is wise not to argue with the patient or attempt to point out the errors of his story. You can always say you disagree with the patient but sympathize with his point of view, or that it may be better to discontinue the discussion until some further time when all persons involved are calmer. Like all displays of tact, there are no hard-and-fast rules, and the nurse must rely on her own good sense and that intangible feeling of working well with persons who are fearful and antagonistic. She must recognize that though antagonism is often expressed toward her, the actual hostility may be intended for another far-distant and frightening person in the patient's personal life, and that sometimes she may have to be a whipping boy for this distant person at whom the patient dare not directly express hostility. She often represents a mother to the patient, and his lies are sometimes the lies of a child who fears punishment from his mother, or fears action contrary to his wants and needs. A calm, pleasant approach and no show of retaliation will give him a feeling of stability and may help him to recognize that there is no need to lie to her. The physician will be doing what he can to help the patient gain a more mature and accurate hold on his emotions, and by working with him the nurse can do much to prevent further emotional turmoil.

Petty Thievery. This is often a problem in working with the very young, with schizophrenics, with the aged, and with luetics. All such persons may be classified as not having learned or not having accepted the theory of "mine and thine." What they see and want, they take. Usually they do not do wrong intentionally. A pretty ribbon, someone's jacket, a bit of jewelry, will appeal to them, and they take it. Sometimes it will be food or some useless object apparently treasured by another patient. Occasionally it will be taken to irritate another patient who is disliked by the petty thief. The great danger in such action lies in the discord it creates, the lost tempers, the actual battles involving other patients, and the ever-present fear that personnel have of being accused of taking patients' valuables. While most hospitals will not allow patients to retain any money or valuable jewelry, some hospitals do feel it is good for the patient to keep his personal belongings which remind him of his home ties and give him the feeling of being a distinct personality. These hospitals will have a clause in the admission blank absolving the hospital from responsibility for loss or theft, but it is the moral responsibility of all staff members to watch those patients who are known to pick up objects belonging to others. Great tact is needed, and, with the very aged, sometimes no more action is necessary than to remove the stolen article quietly and replace it where it belongs. The aged and the luetic have a fairly short memory span and may not even recall taking the article. They tend to hoard all sorts of objects, and it is wise to go through their beds, bureaus, and other possible hiding places regularly, though not at regular times, to look for possible weapons, for articles belonging to others, and for hoarded food.

Patients should know that routine searches are made, and, in the case of a patient who is cognizant of his surroundings, it is wise to let him know when the search is being made. Otherwise, there is a sense of loss of dignity and self-esteem. All of us have many odds and ends of what may appear to be trash to others but mean much to us, and they are often the last little bit of individuality left to the patient. We have no right to intrude upon him and go through these personal items without his knowledge and awareness.

The nurse should take a nonpunitive action, and no retaliation ever should be made when stolen items are found. The doctor will handle the discipline of serious cases of petty thievery. The nurses and attendants have the main task of preventing this by constant watchfulness and tactful guidance of those patients who may pick up interesting and colorful objects. Sometimes the patients who take things need more attention from the staff. Stealing is often a sign of wanting to be loved, of the great need to belong and to have something or someone to belong to you. A happy, busy atmosphere with pleasant surroundings can do much to eliminate stealing.

SUGGESTED REFERENCES

Ballard, L., "Nursing Care of the Schizophrenic," *Trained Nurse & Hospital Review*, 118:252–259, 1947.

De Lourdes, Sister Mary, "Understanding Children," *American Journal of Nursing*, 46:770–772, 1946.

Menninger, Karl A., *The Human Mind*, Alfred A. Knopf, Inc., New York 1942, pp. 372-408.

Menninger, William C., "Psychoneurosis—A Summary for the Nurse," *American Journal of Nursing*, 45:348–350, 1946.

Naranick, Claudia, "The Overactive Patient," *American Journal of Nursing*, 47:97–103, 1947.

Price, Antoinette, "Understanding the Neurotic," *American Journal of Nursing*, 37:878–881, 1937.

Weiss, Madeline O., "Nursing Care of Psychoneurotics," *American Journal of Nursing*, 46:41–42, 1946.

CHAPTER 7

Psychotic Children

BECAUSE IT IS a comparatively new field, and because there is yet so little known about it, we have made a separate chapter about the care of children with emotional disturbances. All small children have emotional upsets accompanying illness, just as adults do. The children discussed in this chapter, however, are those tots diagnosed as actually psychotic. Sometimes the diagnosis will be given in well-known psychiatric terminology; sometimes the term "acute behavior disturbance" will be used. Often these children will be hospitalized "for observation," that tragic phrase which may mean the doctor does not want to label a youngster with the diagnosis of psychosis, or that he is still not sure that the child is really psychotic.

Abnormal Behavior

Since most children are uninhibited little animals at first, how can we tell where a child's behavior stops being normal and becomes abnormal? Almost all children cry, kick, scream, bite, and attack their environment directly when it doesn't give them what they want. Surprisingly early in most infants' lives, however, they learn that a grin, babbling happily, and occasionally changing their minds about a demand will gain the needed attention. Children do more than just *want* attention; they *need* it. It is the most important "vitamin" for growth that is available, and there is no substitute.

Well, some children don't learn how to smile, how to exchange one desire for another, how to respond to affection. Long past infancy, they continue their crying, kicking, biting, or screaming, and they show little effort to try to communicate with others. Sometimes they are mute, and often they are thought to be deaf, until the desperate parents have had all possible tests made and unbelievingly bring the child to the psychiatrist. Frequently, in such a child's history, the mother will make an odd statement: "My baby rejected me almost from his birth." And further study will reveal that these children were often the quiet babies, the so-called "self-sufficient" or unemotional, phlegmatic, cold babies. They rarely cried, and showed little interest in toys, or had only one special toy to which they clung, and mother, or daddy, in a mistaken moment, may have insisted on introducing new toys, which precipitated quite a storm. There seems to be some need for this special toy or loved object; often it is a battered holdover from infancy—a strip of the baby blanket, a soft doll, a pair of discarded woolly slippers—and it cannot be replaced. On admission to the hospital, these little tykes will clutch the dear toy close, clinging to it even at meals and at bathtime. It should not be taken away. As they learn to exchange even the tiniest bit of affection with others—another child in the ward, or a member of the staff—they may seem to discard the toy, but it is always important to them, and, in moments of frustration or hurt, they will seek it out.

I recall one four-year-old whose beloved object—a dirty cylindrical piece of wood—fell behind a well-protected radiator. It landed just beyond reach, and Tommy became literally panic-stricken. His first reaction had seemed to be mere anger, but the squall changed in tone to inconsolable sobbing and screaming, as all of us attempted to retrieve the bit of wood. We tried substitutes, but they were of no value; he wanted this special, precious toy. Even the visitors on the ward helped in our attempt to get behind the radiator, and Tommy quieted a bit as he seemed to sense that we were all trying to return his dearest possession to him. His crying became softer, with little pauses, much like the baby who expects his mother to come after a certain period of crying. It developed a waiting note, and finally, after almost half an hour of prying and poking, we retrieved the object. He seized it quickly, examined it carefully, and became quiet. In a few moments he cast it aside in favor of something else, but he seemed to keep a wary eye on it. Indeed, for weeks, we kept a supply of exact duplicates of the wooden cylinder so there would be no similar panic attacks should one disappear again. This was all a phase in Tommy's hospitalization, but an important one. We can only speculate on what might have happened had we not retrieved his toy; we preferred to instill in him faith and trust in adults, and we feel this was an important first step in his beginning to accept the people around him as a part of the world he could enter trustfully.

These sick youngsters often have a history of extraordinary sensitivity to sound, and frequently show a negative reaction to human speech. Conversely, they are unusually interested in music, and will have favorite records and radio programs, or even may be extraordinarily talented musically. This interest in music and rhythmic sounds and disinterest in speech has led to some interesting hypotheses, one being that music conveys the usual communicating aspects of speech to them, while speech itself is meaningless. The subject has not been studied long enough for any definite conclusions to be drawn, but nurses will do well to remember that a soft, quiet voice will be less apt to cause such children to withdraw from them. A nurse who works with these youngsters will also do well to know many of the rhythm verses of childhood, and be prepared to repeat them hour after hour, or listen to the same record almost unceasingly.

Nursing Techniques

The study of pediatrics teaches very little about how to work with mentally ill children, probably because the fact that children can be psychotic was pretty much ignored until recently. A real effort to make hospital units for disturbed children only has been made in the last decade. How are chil dren psychotic? How can we tell when a child is really ill and not being "naughty"? Psychotic children are examined by pediatricians and sometimes by psychiatrists and, if possible, are treated at home. However, some of these youngsters show no change for the better until they are institutionalized. This is tragic, for children need their own families near them, and most doctors will recommend hospitalization only if the child is so ill that separation from his parents holds less danger than does the lack of institutionalization.

A great many of these children have behavior symptoms which are irritating and baffling: wetting and soiling, muteness, biting, kicking, scratching, stealing, carelessness in dress and in eating, and, in short, all the asocial symptoms which we simply do not accept in our highly socialized life. Taking care of such youngsters is one of the most challenging, fascinating, and frequently disheartening, tasks in nursing. Its rewards are so few and so infrequent that one can easily become discouraged. The nurse has to give and give and give, and few of us are so made that we can continue to give without wanting some return.

Tone of Voice. Since these children do not communicate well, we must consider how to communicate with them. The nurse's voice is of great importance. She doesn't have to have dulcet tones, or a "good" singing voice. The important quality in her voice is genuine affection. Children pick up quickly the real warmth and affection which the nurse can show, even when she must deny the child something he wants immediately. We are not too aware of how our emotions creep into our voices, even when we pride ourselves on our fine control. I recall being busy in the kitchen when a young friend was visiting. My mind was on getting dinner ready, planning for the rest of the day, or similar "important" adult activity. Young Jimmy chattered happily about his latest project—a building venture in the creek on his family's farm—and invited me to join him in it. My answer was, I thought, patient and pleasant, and I was horrified when he looked hurt and said, "You're mad, aren't you? Why?" I put aside my "important" work and sat down to talk over the dam Jimmy was planning, after apologizing for appearing angry. But I have thought about it a great deal. The boy and I were close friends and had shared many happy hours identifying insects and birds, working in the garden, or just rambling through the countryside. Why had I been angry, or at least annoyed to the point that he could pick up the tone in my voice? Heretofore, I had shown great interest in the dam; I had willingly "gotten down to his level" in our many excursions, but in the instance cited above I had felt that he was intruding in my adult world, and my voice showed it.

The sigh of impatience we think we have suppressed, the little edginess of irritation, the sharpened pitch when we have been frightened—these show in our voices, and children, especially these sick children, seem to be acutely sensitive to them.

The Child's Level. Carrying this thought further, watch adults out with children and notice the tendency to accept children for a short while but then brusquely to abandon them for a more adult level of enjoyment. It isn't easy to play, or work, with children eight hours a day, but we can make it easier by not setting up adult standards and limits for children. We can enjoy being at the child's level, if we let him know, and if we know, that there is also an adult level to which we must return occasionally, but that there is no special dividing line which the child cannot cross. He will learn to be an adult by imitating adult behavior, so, for his sake, we cannot stay constantly at the child's level. I am purposely stressing this matter of levels. For levels there are, but the way we approach them is important. Rather than accept levels as neatly defined and fenced sections of growth, why not accept the child for what he is—a person with some limitations owing to his lack of experience in our society? As adults, we can help them gain social experience without frustrating them. Taking small children on trips—in town, to the zoo, or across the country—is an interesting example. So often we see parents with their youngsters trying to force the two- or three-year-old and somewhat older children to conform to adult standards,

PSYCHOTIC CHILDREN

largely because they fear the embarrassment of the child's uncluttered, and at times alarmingly direct, approach to matters we tend to cover up. How often do parents try to hush children in restaurants or on the streetcar? Notice the slightly amused, withal embarrassed, faces of parents whose child says loudly, "Why is that lady wearing such a funny hat?" "Isn't this a dirty old bus?" "I have to go to the toilet." With a bit of courage, most of us can answer these questions in an ordinary tone, and the matter is settled without upsetting the child or setting up ridiculous taboos. At the most, the parent may have a fleeting embarrassment with the strangers who listen in, but the chances are they will never see them again, and aren't their children of greater importance than strangers?

Concept of Time. There are many things to take into consideration in working with young children. Time is endless to them; it has no great meaning and tomorrow, or later, is something they cannot grasp. Try to plan your day beforehand so you can help them with concrete time sections. *"Now* is when we eat breakfast; then after breakfast we wash our hands and play in the sandbox." Or, with the child who can understand the figures on a clock: "Now we are going to finger paint; when the big hand stands up straight and the little hand is right there (and make it a definite spot), we shall go for a walk." "If we take our lollipops out of our mouths and wave them around, they get taken away"—and if you make some such warning, don't abruptly snatch away the lollipops (children will take them out to see how they change in size or color), but warn again "I see a lollipop being waved." Usually such an approach results in a giggle, and the candy goes back in the mouth. Try to think as the child does, in concrete, small time sequences, with every new experience filled with wonder and curiosity and a little fear. Accept the child for what he is, and recognize his limitations. Prepare him to accept adult standards by making them interesting and fun.

Reconciling Standards of Children and Adults. Not too long ago, I took two small girls across the country. They were four and five years old, and very charming travel companions.

We took five dolls, and several comic books, and a couple of lollipops tucked in my purse for a surprise. There were also an old handkerchief and some rubber bands; I have learned to carry these with me to make all sorts of dolls and animals; it amuses small children for hours. Our trip was uneventful. That is, there were no especially embarrassing moments, and the children were quite well-behaved, so the passengers and hostess on the plane told me, in tones of wonder. I take only small credit for it; the children had been told we were to take this trip, and I made it a point to visit with them on the whole long journey, and to answer their questions fully and honestly. When the bigger one said she didn't want to be strapped in her seat, I pointed to the lights telling about fastening seat belts and explained, "When that light goes on, everyone fastens the seat belts; when the one next to it goes on, I'll have to put out my cigarette." She became quite interested in watching for the light and told me eagerly when to put out my cigarette. Turn about was fair play; I had told her when to fasten her seat belt. We had no difficulty with seat belts after that; she and her sister watched for the lights eagerly, and a number of the passengers waited with amusement, and I think some pleasure, to hear them sing out, "It's time to fasten your seat belt." We played with the dolls for a while, I read to them, and they were quite agreeable when I said I was tired and maybe they would like to entertain themselves for a while. We took turns being politely entertaining to each other, and much as I would have enjoyed some adult conversation, I gave all my attention to the children. On pondering this, I came to the conclusion that too often we adults want only to be entertained by children but are not willing to entertain them. We casually join them when it suits us, instead of courteously inviting them to join us, or asking permission to join them. We intrude on them because they are smaller and less knowing than we, and we feel that it is our right as adults. We also seem to feel that it is only our interest which matters when we are with children. That is what I mean about disliking the matter of getting down to their level.

Rather, we should plan our time so that the children have a real—rather than casual—role in our life with them.

Once I congratulated a friend for her two charming children, one fifteen years old and one twenty. I was particularly impressed by the fifteen-year-old boy, who was polite, friendly, and unobtrusive, and a highly intelligent conversationalist. My friend was surprised at my compliment and said, "But we've always treated the children like any other members of the family with individual patterns." How many families do that? I fear that too often the adults in the family expect a child to conform to a precut pattern, based on strange mixtures of Victorian ideals and the hopes and dreams of the parents who feel that their own childhoods lacked something and they must make life different for their children. This is a dangerous trap into which the nurse may fall without thought. She will try to work on the children's unit with her preconceived ideas of child behavior, colored by her own background, the smattering of pediatric nursing she had as a student, and what intellectualization she can make of her own emotions. I'm afraid she will forget that children are individuals, each with a personality distinct and different from every other child, and that each child has not only the right but the need to be an individual, accepted for what he is.

As such, children are entitled to the respect and courtesy one gives to any other human being. The child's small size and lack of social sophistication tends to make adults treat him with amused condescension or as a plaything. Children are neither; they are growing individual persons, and their needs and wants are basically the same as those of adults; they differ only in their ability to interpret these needs adequately or in a socially acceptable manner.

We must remember many small, important things when we work with children, one of which is an actual physical difference in the point of view. Kneel down to a child's height occasionally; the world looks different from there, especially the indoor world of adult-sized furniture and utilities. And kneel down, if you will, to a child's height in thought and action. Children see many things we do not notice from our height, or because we take them for granted. They are rather new to a world filled with many things, and they are curious about what they see. I am sure the "destructiveness" of many small children is not conscious destructiveness as much as curiosity about what makes things work, how they are put together, what will happen if that interesting screw is removed. From their height, the nuts, bolts, screws, and working parts of much household paraphernalia are temptingly near and need to be explored. Purses are filled with so many things that attract a child: shiny lipsticks and compacts, mirrors, money (which is fun because it jingles), handkerchiefs, and all sorts of things. And what a fuss adults make when the child does get into a purse, or pulls apart the furniture. Of course, we cannot condone such behavior, but we can substitute pull-apart toys, and old purses and compacts, so the child can satisfy his curiosity without damaging something valuable. Most important, we can divert his attention without making a perfectly natural curiosity seem naughty. The scolding and hand slapping may, in the long run, prove more damaging to a child's growth than the monetary damage to personal property is worth. It's a thought to consider seriously.

A Positive Approach. Well, how do we meet this curiosity in the child, this need for growth and exploration in an adult world? For one thing, let's find some substitute for "No, no." Is there a positive way to approach the child who is doing something which is forbidden him, or is dangerous? There is, if we stop to consider it. We can substitute, "Let's go see where the book about the doggy is" for "Tommy, put that magazine back; don't tear it; give the doll to Susan." We can say, with good humor in our voice, "This is strictly forbidden for small fry" and get a co-operative response, where, "No, no, you're too small to do that" will only move the child to prove he can too do it. It isn't easy to substitute positive suggestions when your whole being wants to scream out an irritated "Stop it this instant." But it gets to be rather fun to see how often we can avoid the negative approach, and the response of the children is so much quicker and easier that it is worth the effort. On the other hand, are we never to let the children see that something has made us angry? Must we hide our emotions? The answer to that is "No." The child fears the person who shows no emotional response more than the one who responds overemotionally. The main thing is to respond to a child's activity naturally and without feeling uneasy about how you respond. If you are angry, it's perfectly legitimate, and you can tell the child you were angry, but that you still love him. Too often, anger means rejection, and it's rather sad to grow up thinking that when the people we love are angry with us they no longer love us. It isn't true, usually; it's rather difficult to have an emotion as strong as anger toward someone for whom we have no affection.

I recall playing with a couple of four-year-olds one day. I sat on the bench while the children played busily with seesaws and climbing equipment. Eventually they climbed up on me, which was an acceptable and a rather regular practice. Little Mary began to play with my hair. She dearly loved to comb hair, and usually I let her comb mine, but this day I was irritable and didn't want my hair mussed, and said, "Don't comb my hair, Mary. I don't want it combed." She stopped at once and said, "You don't love me." My negative approach had gotten me into this, and I gathered her into my lap to explain that I did love her, even though I had forbidden her to comb my hair. There were other things we could do together, I suggested, and after some little time spent in just holding her close, she accepted a substitute activity. The next morning Mary told me not to comb her hair; she didn't want it combed. I acceded. She had as much right as I to not want her hair combed that day. Somewhat later in the day, she was ready to have her hair brushed and combed so we could go for a walk, and no further reactions to my original refusal to have her comb my hair were shown.

Routines. The preceding discussion has led us to one of the biggest problems of a psychiatric children's ward: How much routine is necessary? Is it really vital that children brush their teeth, wash their faces and hands, have their hair combed? Certainly with these disturbed children it is not. Isn't it more important to have a child who feels comfortable and at ease than an uneasy and disturbed child whose hair is neat and hands are clean? Comfortable emotions are so much more important than looking nice. Dr. Alice Keliher has said, and wisely, "Never does a child need love more than when he is at his unloveliest." And never is it more difficult to love a child than when he is untidy, soiled, or hostile. It takes a great deal of fortitude to reach out with warmth and love on so many occasions.

Then are there to be no routines? Oh, yes; we need the routines, and so do the children. We need a framework of washing, eating, and sleeping times, but we can be flexible within that framework. Not everyone who works with these children agrees on the matter of routines, and I express my own ideas because I find I can work better within a framework of routines. When I can work more easily, the children respond more readily. Again, it's a matter of finding where we are most comfortable and working at that level, and to the very best of our ability. I do feel that a child needs some boundaries, or he becomes frightened. Unlimited freedom can be most terrifying, and few adults, let alone children, can accept it. But within the defined boundaries we can be very relaxed indeed. We can say comfortably, "Well, we usually wash our hands before we eat because clean hands are nice, but you don't have to wash them. Philip is ready to wash his, though, I see." Rarely will all the children rebel against a given routine at the same time, and the mere fact of another's conformation will often bring a young rebel to the point of conforming too. It is wise to accept this with no comment.

The one routine which all can rebel against at once is bedtime. It takes very little to turn the quiet prebedtime hour into a literal madhouse, and it is one of the most difficult things to halt until there have been tears, tantrums, and several kicked shins. Keep bedtime as quietly cheerful as possible, nip in the bud attempts at hilarity, even if it means banishing one or more of the children to another room, "so the children who are ready to sleep can go to sleep." Away from the stimulation of the other youngsters, the rebel often gives up to the genuine tiredness he feels. Occasionally, he may be so stimulated that he needs to have an adult with him who will keep him from injury. He may need to be alone in a room with a book, or a small phonograph to play softly. He may need to be held, firmly and quietly, in your lap. Isolation from the other children will keep him from stimulating them and from learning the tremendous power he has to upset the whole ward. Power to a child is a magic and fearful thing, and his use of it without restraint is terrifying. That is one reason a structured situation is needed, so that the child has some boundaries, even though he may stretch them and break them at times.

Love as Therapy. It seems to me that the most important thing we can teach the emotionally disturbed child is that we love him, and we must say so in words and actions over and over again. Dr. Levy tells the story of his wife's feeling sure her mother didn't love her when she was small because she never *made* her do her homework, while other parents did. Just such small things are misinterpreted by children, and they quickly learn to expect correction and punishment from the persons who love them. The nurse is a parent surrogate, and she must correct her charges often, but loss of love should never be inferred from her admonishments. If something has annoyed you, don't try to hide it; if you are amused when the mashed potatoes fly across the table, laugh. But be ready to explain that certain behavior isn't accepted by most people and that you still love Johnny, even when you must restrict his behavior.

Sometimes we are careless about our affection and use it as a weapon with children (and with adults too). We say in effect, and sometimes in so many words, "I won't love you if you do that," or "People don't like little girls who pick their noses," or some similar threatening phrase. And how cruel it is to promise withdrawal of the most necessary part of a child's life. With these sick children, the nurse must say again and again, in words and by her actions, "I love you; I don't like the thing you just did, but I love you." She must be able to pick up an untidy, hostile child, and keep him from hurting another child, her, or himself, and help him feel that she is not rejecting him. There are no specific directions for doing this. Far wiser people than I have foundered in an attempt to teach men to love one another, but if you genuinely "like" children, you should have no trouble learning what is the right reaction in a given situation.

There are other more tangible problems of caring for these youngsters. One of the simplest, and most irritating, is their apparent lack of ability to perform the acts of keeping clean—using the toilet properly, washing their hands, brushing their teeth. Since we nurses have been taught the almost holy ritual of keeping clean (we do say it is next to godliness), we tend to overstress these acts, especially with the child who does not perform them when he appears big enough to know how. We must keep reminding ourselves that these children are sick. There is some reason behind the soiling, the extreme disinterest in, or even fear of, washing. And we must school ourselves to accept the child, even when he is not too tidy. It is not easy, but once he learns that he is accepted for himself, he may be ready to give a little something to you—washing his hands before meals, or using the toilet. That is really a gift; the child has given up a practice he enjoyed for something less enjoyable because he likes you. Accept it humbly and without much fuss, but enjoy it for what it represents—one move in the direction of his making a positive contact with another human being. I remember, with the same glow of satisfaction I felt then, the first time one of our most silent and rebellious four-year-olds kissed me. It was a very hesitant kiss, given quite gravely, and followed by ignoring me for a while. After months of being bitten, this was a complete and wonderful change, which I accepted as a gift, thanking Hank for it gravely. For days I felt as if a halo were glowing right above my head. And this one, tiny step forward did mark a change in young Hank's behavior.

There was no magic change into a "normal" little boy, and he is still hospitalized, but he began to give a little more, to come spontaneously to the staff members, to seize their hands, and to smile up at them. He was finally beginning to trust other human beings. If you get discouraged at working with psychotic adults, your heart will break working with these children, but the satisfactions are great, even though they are rare and slow in appearing.

Patience. The nurse will need a degree of patience accorded only to saints to meet some of the daily events of a psychotic children's unit. Johnny will flood the bathroom five times a day; as often, the plumber will grumble about having to make repairs; Timmy will defecate in some hidden corner of the playroom, and Debbie will play in the feces before you have found it; Mark will hit Janie with a wooden toy, and have a real, screaming tantrum when you pick her up to comfort her; Jimmy will drop a favorite toy in an inaccessible place and have a panic reaction with unconsolable sobbing when it cannot be rescued. The dietitian will be horror-stricken because an eight-year-old has eaten five eggs for breakfast, though the pediatrician has assured her and you that nothing dire will come of it. Mary will demand the same thing to eat morning, noon, and night for three weeks, and the pantry girl will try to coax her to eat something else, though you have left express orders to let Mary eat what she wants.

You see, what happens in each case is that you, and all the others who work with you, will judge for the child—will make decisions for him—and that is not good. Mary may be sick and tired of the same food, but some inner need we do not yet understand makes her demand it; when that need is satisfied, she will give it up, and her physical health will not have been greatly impaired. On the other hand, if some food habit, some lack of social training, does not come up to expected standards for normal children, is it more important to have a physically normal child, who complies with our ideals of the healthy child, or a more nearly emotionally normal child, with some slight physical handicap?

Attitudes and Psychotic Children. So far, I have really said very little about attitudes in caring for these children. They are the same attitudes we use for adults, the same attitudes we use in all our daily living, but they must be used far more judiciously. The one thing these youngsters never get enough of is love—love unsolicited, daily and constantly, even when we must deny them something. Children need some boundaries to their world, some limits which tell them we are protecting them. We must learn to say "No," quietly, calmly, and unflinchingly. At the same time, we must be ready to substitute something positive for the denial which was necessary. Sometimes, if the child shows a proclivity for choosing only dangerous activities, such as chewing electric wires, putting metal objects into wall plugs, and playing with bits of sharp glass or metal, we must guard against these hazards with all the safety devices we can command, *but* we must make the safe things so attractive that the child will learn to prefer them. Even though we must deny, we must try to avoid saying "No" as often as possible. Practice saying "You can't do this," without saying "No, no." It is difficult at first, but playing a game with it will make you remarkably facile at this useful ability. When the playroom is in a shambles, and the children seem on the verge of exploding all over the place, try saying, "How would you like to go for a walk?" (or play with clay, or go outdoors) or anything available in your particular hospital to take the children away from the disturbed—and disturbing —room; children don't like untidiness in great quantity. If possible, all units for disturbed children should have more than one playroom so that someone can tidy up the disordered room while the children are in another. Tidying up is an endless job on such units, but it is vital. The children have a difficult enough time keeping their small, topsy-turvy world in any sort of alignment; if their surroundings are awry, they have even greater difficulty.

Attitudes are most important in working with these children. Their extreme sensitivity to the nurse's emotional response to them tends to create a defensiveness in the nurses, so a vicious circle is started. The first rule, which is the same as the first rule of caring for all people, is to be natural. Children are natural because they have not yet learned all the layers of "civilized unnaturalness" which make up modern people. These children express their aggression freely, and their love can be expressed just as freely when they know what love is; both these emotions can be overwhelming. The nurse must, in short, be prepared to see naked emotions and must be able to meet them with warmth, understanding, and relaxation. The psychotic child has fewer layers of civilization, has learned less of the social amenities, and has little or no storehouse of remembered "social graces." Because of the latter situation, the nurse does not lead such children *back* to acceptable behavior as she does with adults; rather, she must teach such behavior, and teach it so that the child wants to be like other children. It is a long, slow process.

Emotional Entanglements

There are many problems for the nurse caring for autistic or psychotic youngsters, not the least of which is the emotional entanglement she can get into, both with the children themselves and with the parents. The emotions are quite different, for the nurse may soon lose herself in giving affection to the children but may become quite hostile to the parents. She may blame the parent for the child's illness. It is true that something in the home background and emotional life may have caused the child's illness, but we dare not become moralistic and judgmental about this. First of all, we know all too little about why these things happen, and second—and I think this is something we gloss over at times—the parents do not deliberately set out to reject their child, to dislike him, or to be cruel to him. They are merely acting as individuals who have become parents, under emotional pressures and needs of their own, and often they operated to the best of their ability.

Perhaps some parents perform a poor best, but we don't blame people for having arthritis or a cardiac condition, so why should we blame them for having personalities which seem to make them poor parents?

Another way of looking at this is to remember that the ideal "good" parent is based on rather artificial standards, which we have set up according to the individual reactions we have to our own childhoods, to our own parents, and to the things they did with which we didn't agree. Is there anyone reading this chapter who hasn't said to himself, many years ago, "When I grow up I won't make my children go to bed when they don't want to," or, "When I grow up I won't make my children wash their hands, or come in from play because it's nap time," or any one of a dozen minor rebellions against restrictions and standards? These are the somewhat unrealistic standards we use when we become judgmental about the parents of the sick children. Accept them for themselves, and above all, remember that they are frightened and worried to death about these children and their own mixed-up emotions concerning the hospitalization. They need reassurance and friendliness, and much help when their child shows an affection for the nurse which the parents feel rightfully belongs to them.

Take time to visit with the parents, if they seem to desire this; take time to show them the unit, the things their child has done, and plans for the child's day; take time to arrange for the parents to see the doctor or the social worker if they seem to need such a visit. Include the parents in your thinking about the child and his future, for the final disposition of the child, whether he improves, recovers, or must be institutionalized for life, is up to the parents, and they will need a great deal of help with all of these problems.

Another danger in this nursing field is the great attachment which the nurse may make to the children. Yes, we want nurses to love these sick kids, to hold them, pet them, play with them. But the nurse must not let herself become so involved with them that they become her only life. She will be tempted time and again to buy a toy for Susie, or a book for Johnny, or a dress for the orphaned child who has no family. We must think carefully before we start any of these activities, and determine the real reason for doing them, which will prove to be, quite often, because of the personal pleasure the nurse receives from presenting these gifts and watching the child's face light up. This happens often and is so common that we may fail to see the dangers inherent in the practice, ignoring the factors leading to children's hospitalization. For it isn't fair to Susie or Johnny to make either one your pet; you may leave the hospital employ quite suddenly; you may marry and have a child of your own; you may become ill. Any one of a dozen things can happen which will take you away from the children you have taught to depend entirely upon you, and when that happens, it is the child who suffers and who has one more trauma to overcome.

Despite the somewhat threatening note I've added here, work with these sick children is fun and satisfying. Every day more is being learned about why these youngsters become psychotic, and the outlook is a bit more hopeful for them. It is a highly specialized aspect of nursing, and additional education is required for the nurse who wishes to make the field her specialty, but it is extremely worth while.

SUGGESTED REFERENCES

Bettelheim, Bruno, *Love Is Not Enough,* The Free Press, Glencoe, Ill., 1950.

Colm, Hanna, "Play as a Means of Communication between Child and Adult," *The Journal of Child Psychiatry,* 2:100–112, 1951.

Freud, A., and Burlingham, D. T., *Infants without Families,* International Universities Press, Inc., New York, 1944, pp. 56–100.

Greenberg, Harold A., *et al., Child Psychiatry in the Community,* G. P. Putnam's Sons, New York, 1950.

Josselyn, Irene M., *Psychosocial Development of Children,* Family Service Association of America, New York, 1948, pp. 7–20.

Levy, John, and Munroe, Ruth, *The Happy Family,* Alfred A. Knopf, Inc., New York, 1950, pp. 240–319.

CHAPTER 8

Love, the Basis of Attitude Therapy

LOVE HAS COME to mean so many things to each of us that we find it difficult to put this feeling into words. The dictionary tells us that love is "to regard with a strong feeling of affection; to have a devoted attachment to." How then, you ask, can we use this strong feeling in the treatment of the mentally ill? We can supply a number of humanity's many needs easily and with no great effort on our part. Today's children are better fed, better clothed, and better housed than they have been for centuries. Unfortunately, in supplying these physical comforts, we have stressed efficiency, scientific factual knowledge, and mechanical works more than the less tangible things. We speak glibly of security for children, and assume that good nourishing food, a clean place to sleep, and freedom from physical want will assure healthy adults, yet our population shows a frightening increase in the rate of mental illness. Although some of this increase is due to the tendency to compute more statistics, and more accurate statistics, and to better methods of diagnosis, much of the increase is due, too, to the great pressure under which we now live. In simplifying our physical lives, we have mechanized them. We become too busy pushing buttons, polishing the tile and chromium, or measuring pills and vitamins, to give time for companionship's sake, to give the warmth of spirit and interest in individuals which is vitally, if immeasurably, important.

I'm sure that nurses (though the fault lies not only with them) would cheerfully carry out a doctor's order to cuddle a sick baby for fifteen minutes every two hours, or even to spend half an hour twice a day reading to an elderly bedridden patient, but patients, being people, don't want cuddling or reading by the clock. We must be prepared to give affection, or attention, or love (it is all the same thing in intent) when the person needs it, and we fail rather often because giving love is difficult. When it becomes an order, we tend to rebel. "I can't like everybody," the young nurse says, and we agree. But we can't avoid everyone we dislike, and the next best thing is to face that fact and then try to approach these patients with at least normal courtesy. Strangely, courtesy may alter the person we dislike, and we find that he isn't so bad after all. Even if we don't, we feel a little glow of pride which is better than the feeling of anger with ourselves, often based on guilt, which we experience when we express only unadulterated annoyance with someone. Our society makes so many demands upon us to hide emotions which are negative that when we do feel them, they are usually accompanied by guilt, which, in turn, makes us feel uncomfortable and more hostile.

This is not intended to foster any Pollyanna-like regard for people—for Pollyannas fool no one, not even themselves—but rather to foster an interest in individuals for the individual's sake. Interest need not always be based on affection or even fondness, but interest in people is rather like a chain reaction, creating wider and wider interests and making work fun instead of drudgery. We all want people to be interested in us; it raises our self-esteem, makes us feel that we have some purpose. And the crossest or most unreachable patient begins to react favorably when he recognizes that you are interested in him. He has a little bit of faith in himself again, and that tiny morsel of self-respect, or esteem, or dignity, can be the vital spark in resocialization or rehabilitation, or just in getting the patient to become one of us again.

Rejection

In reviewing the causative factors in mental illness, research workers have come up again and again with the main fact that the mentally ill withdraw from society or fight societal rules because they feel rejected—not one of the group. Each person reacts according to his own basic personality pattern, but the cause is often, if not always, the feeling of not truly belonging. How do we know we "belong" to the group in which we are placed? What gives us the feeling of not belonging? The infant soon learns he is loved by the comforts he receives from those around him, and later by the smiles, attention, and affection which he gets. He learns to earn that love, first by his smiles and cooing, then by his other more co-ordinated actions, by following within his personal limits the patterns of behavior set up for him by his parent surrogates. Thus he earns the love, affection, or pleasant attention of his group. As he progresses to school and then to work, he gets attention from the secondary groups (of which there are many) into which he is drawn by his activities through conforming to the group's pattern of behavior in given situations. Each group has its own pattern, largely following a rough plan of a leader, and some type of regulations to keep the group cohesive. The mentally ill find they cannot fit into a certain group, or any group. No matter what the rules may be, someone, or the group itself, fails to give all the attention which is needed to keep the sick person functioning comfortably within that group, and because this frightens or angers him, he reacts either by withdrawing or by fighting. The latter is achieved by deliberately flouting group regulations.

The Hospital Group

Once in the hospital, the sick person finds himself in a different sort of group. Its center of cohesion lies in its being made up of members of society like himself, persons who have difficulty in fitting into groups. Its leaders are usually well members of society with understanding and knowledge, persons who can meet the varied and sometimes strange behavior of individual members of that group without causing the individual to feel he is rejected or must withdraw from this one last social group with which he may identify. The nurse

LOVE, THE BASIS OF ATTITUDE THERAPY

is the leader of such groups of sick persons by reason of her constant attendance and her close contact with the members. Hers is the task of making the patient feel that he is a worthwhile member of society, and her basic tool is love or understanding, or giving attention, while gently helping these bewildered and frightened persons to follow the really simple standards of group behavior. That is why we say love is the basis of attitude therapy.

The nurse and adjunctive workers must feel some warmth for their fellow men, must be capable of giving attention in the most adverse circumstances, and of utilizing each tiny step forward which the individual patient makes, while keeping the entire group of patients in their care within the limits of safety and social requirements. Courtesy is the first step, and the easiest to take. It is simply being polite to others in all circumstances, regarding every individual as a fellow human being worthy of feeling some self-esteem. Persons so treated react almost automatically by behaving like persons of some esteem. Stripped of his self-respect, any person will do and say things he could not do if he had a feeling that someone—any one person—felt he was an individual and therefore worthy. Courtesy then requires that we call patients by their full names with a title, that we respect them according to their individual achievements in life, no matter under what circumstances we meet them in the hospital. For all our closeness to patients we are strangers to them, and they are rightfully resentful of being called by their given names or a nickname which may be distasteful to them, or a nickname which may reflect a state of life they do not care to acknowledge. Patients in psychiatric hospitals are in a peculiarly helpless state to do anything about their treatment, and because of this we have the responsibility of seeing that their treatment is above reproach. Once patients find themselves being met with respect, courtesy, and affection, they respond because they cannot help but respond. Each person may take a different length of time to make that response, but he *will* respond. Dr. Karl Menninger puts it simply and beautifully, "If we can love:—This is the touchstone. This is the key to all the therapeutic program of the modern psychiatric hospital; it dominates the behavior of its staff from the director down to the gardener."

SUGGESTED REFERENCES

Bennett, A. M., "Psychiatric Nursing," *American Journal of Nursing,* 39:395–400, 1939.

The Bible: the Old and New Testaments.

Gibran, Kahlil, *The Prophet,* Alfred A. Knopf, Inc., New York, 1944.

Liebman, Joshua L., *Peace of Mind,* Simon and Schuster, New York, 1946.

Menninger, Karl A., *Love against Hate,* Harcourt, Brace and Company, Inc., New York, 1942, pp. 260–294.

CHAPTER 9

The Nurse as an Individual

THE COMPLEX REASONS young people have for entering nursing are numerous and range from the conscious to the deep unconscious needs of the individual. Usually we have formed an ideal about the figure of the nurse, and we imagine a role which we attempt to meet. This role depicts a person serving humanity by taking care of those members of the group who need help in recuperating from a physical illness or trauma, or by being a mother, feeding, bathing, and otherwise caring for a helpless, childlike person. Early in our careers we discover that illness and trauma are accompanied by psychological changes enhancing the nurse's mother role. To attain the goal we set for ourselves, we learn the workings of the wonderful mechanism of the human body and the many ways that mechanism may go awry, as well as what we can do to assist the traumatized machinery to function on a new compromise level which may be temporary or permanent.

A tremendous amount of knowledge with an accompanying responsibility is given nurse students in a comparatively short time. It is a responsibility which forces the roles of a mature, capable "mother" figure upon us, even if we do not consciously accept being mothers. We learn that we must meet the needs of each patient, assist the doctor in his work, keep numerous records, teach and guide auxiliary personnel, maintain an efficiently run unit, and act as hostess and interpreter to the patients' families and visitors. For a time, we are lost as individuals, by virtue of the uniform, the rigidity of our training, and our own bewilderment at the many demands made upon us. As we gain security in our knowledge, dovetailing this with reality problems, we begin to emerge as individuals again; that is, we become a compound of our own ideals of a nurse, plus the school's ideals, plus the public's ideals. We become nurses—persons in uniform, having a defined body of knowledge and skills, certified by law, molded by public opinion, and often lost as individuals. Recent studies by a sociologist reveal a threefold stereotype of the nurse, not always flattering. Summed up roughly, this stereotype shows a nurse to be a paid public servant, with a great deal of knowledge of "forbidden" facts of life, and a job consisting of unpleasant and semiskilled or skilled tasks. The key words in the picture are probably "paid, public servant," with all the connotations the various social levels of the public put upon the word "servant." The implication is there: we are paid for service, and service is expected of us. It is our responsibility to make of that service a dignified act of helpfulness and courtesy. Service does not mean degradation or a lower caste; most of us function better in our complex society when we serve, whether this means being a clerk or an executive or a housewife.

Responsibility to One's Self

The foregoing facts place a grave responsibility upon the nurse who wishes to retain some individuality. Perhaps the most difficult lesson for the young nurse to learn is to meet the demands of the public while satisfying her own needs and desires. As a student, she gives up many of the pleasures and freedoms of her nonnurse friends. Just as they are emerging into the adult world, earning money, meeting young men, and enjoying their first independence as members of adult society, the student nurse is isolated from more normal social life, spends long hours in study and hard work, and has most restricted hours and very little income. Early in her career the nurse becomes "different" from the friends of her childhood and adolescence. Although much of the difference may be due to the strictness of nursing schools (even in these days of increased freedom), a large part of it is the knowledge the student nurse is acquiring. Friends and family are eager to share these experiences in studies and work, they ask numerous questions which put an even greater burden upon the student as she attempts to meet their demands for a person with unending knowledge about the human body. With this new knowledge she has the pressure of awareness that a human life may depend upon her newly acquired actions and knowledge.

All this responsibility is apt to make us overlook an important point in our development—a responsibility to ourselves. We must retain a certain amount of animal selfishness or become so lost in a narrow world of efficiency, dexterity, and perfection of function that we emerge as mechanical persons without much feeling for our fellow human beings. One *must* have some interest in self to understand others, to empathize with and assist others with a real understanding of human needs rather than a knowledge of physical mechanics alone.

Many schools have adopted well-rounded programs of social life, but the individual nurse must take action. If she has a hobby, she should continue with it or adopt new hobbies. Interest in the world about her should increase as she becomes aware of herself as a citizen. Because of her peculiar maturity, and because of society's need for nursing services, she should be preparing herself for a life with many facets. Today, the married nurse and the nurse with children are being accepted on many hospital staffs, and this mixture of careers demands a wide range of interests and activities. The nurse's family will soon grow weary of just hospital news and bits about newly acquired nursing knowledge; they will expect, as she should expect of herself, that she know something of world events and how they will affect her and her family; that she be aware of the theater, the sports world, the many arts, and the wide range of interests most persons have. Paradoxically, the wider our interests (unless we try to encompass too much, of course), the greater our knowledge is in our own field and the more successful is our practice. Look about you: the most popular nurses with patients and staff are usually those who chat easily and readily about gardening, painting, knitting, world affairs, the baseball scores, etc. They have accepted the role of the nurse and have woven into it their own personalities, emerging as individuals. This is the responsibility of each nurse, and until she manages to do this she is failing herself. It is only as individuals that we can take our place in society.

Responsibility to Society

We mentioned earlier that the nurse is a paid public servant, that society places her in that position, and that she herself has had a little to do with creating that role. Public service is a pretty all-inclusive word and can be frightening. Just what does it entail? From personal experience, I know that the first years of nursing give one the feeling of doing good, and we tend to give ourselves shiny halos, feeling pretty smug about our places in the world. Reality comes to each of us in a different way. For some, the harsh impact of reality is in the first contact with death; others find it in the first birth witnessed; for many, it is in caring for a tragically wasting illness and lingering death in a person of promise. Our reactions vary, and the halo may tarnish considerably as we begin to recognize that a nurse must know more than how to give physical care to the sick. Patients' families, the community, and our own families turn to us for advice and suggestions. The pressure of what we are in the eyes of the public helps form our own idea of nursing, and it is not always a happy picture. Society is pretty diverse and pretty demanding, and we must meet those demands, varied as they are.

Mr. R. L. Birdwhistell of the Sociology Department, University of Louisville, interviewed a number of persons (patients, doctors, nonpatients, nurses, and students) in the Louisville area, the hill district of Kentucky, Columbus, rural Ohio, and Chicago to learn what a cross section of society

THE NURSE AS AN INDIVIDUAL

thinks a nurse is. While this was a limited survey, it serves to point out some of the demands and shows how a sample of the public felt about nursing and nurses. It is cited here because it is realistic and objective and may help the individual nurse to accept her role in society by better understanding what that role is. Very briefly reviewed, and lifted from the context of the entire paper, the nurse is thought of as a skilled *or* semi-skilled person having *close relationships* with the persons in her care. While there was no mention made of meeting the psychological needs of the patient, this was implied in the expectation of her meeting *all* the patient's needs—being a warm, understanding, and knowledgeable person. Service, with its connotations dependent upon the social level of the persons interviewed, ranged from a semiskilled servant to a skilled technician who knew all about everything. Certainly if the nurse is to attain the skill and knowledge needed to meet daily the demands of sick persons from all social groups, she must look beyond the present rather narrow limits of the nursing school itself. She will have to do much of the seeking for further knowledge on her own, but because her work is so closely interwoven with the life of the community, she should be guided to seek further education in the field of the social sciences. This does not mean she must go to school for the rest of her life, though learning does not stop with the attainment of a degree or a diploma. It does suggest that she investigate courses in the fields of sociology, psychology, social anthropology, and social psychology. Such courses are available in practically all colleges, and while the nurse may have no desire or need for attaining a degree, the extra classes, the contacts with persons outside the limits of her discipline, and the stimulation of added knowledge will make her a person better able to fill her role in society, *and to enjoy herself while doing so.*

For the nurse who finds such schoolwork of no interest, there are night classes in local high schools for all sorts of interesting hobbies from leathercraft to voice training. These lead to new friendships, new group contacts, and a better, if informal, sociological background. She soon finds that nursing is a role which she can never drop entirely, whether or not she leaves the field to follow other life plans. Neighbors and acquaintances will seek her out in times of trouble, and the better her understanding of people, the better she can meet their needs. She will utilize her knowledge and skills in every walk of life, in every role, and the broader her background in the social sciences, the better she will be able to co-ordinate her skills and knowledge to satisfy her own needs as well as society's demands.

You will notice that the bibliographies in this book are rather brief, and do not nearly cover the field of psychiatry or psychiatric nursing. This has been done intentionally. First of all, it is my hope that all of my readers will have learned how to use a library by now, and searching in a library on your own is an excellent exercise, promoting growth and a liberal mind much more than does looking to the end of a chapter for further reading suggestions. Second, I fear that some of the books I should like to list here would startle many nursing instructors and cause great wonderment among the students. Since I emphasize the nurse as an individual, I should like you to read the great books of all time, dip into the philosophies of the Old World, of the eighteenth century especially, read the first novelists (after all, the novel is a very new form of literature), ponder the descriptions of persons written by the "good" authors of the past two centuries. You will learn much of psychiatric principles from such reading, and you will learn a great deal more about people than you can from sticking to textbooks and specialized journals. Since psychiatry is that medical specialty dealing with mental disorders, get an over-all view of people and life as the great writers have portrayed these for us; then you will be able to study the deviations with a clearer idea of what is deviate. Your faith may be shaken at times, but a stronger faith will emerge, and a truer one, for by judicious reading about man you cannot help but come away awed with the truly wonderful creation he is.

SUGGESTED REFERENCES

Beard, Mary, "Creative Nursing," *American Journal of Nursing,* 36:69, 1936.

Birdwhistell, R. L., "Social Science and Nursing Education: Some Tentative Suggestions," *Fifty-fifth Annual Report,* National League of Nursing Education, New York, 1949, pp. 315–328.

Menninger, Karl A., *The Human Mind,* Alfred A. Knopf, Inc., New York, 1942, pp. 408–410.

Weiss, M. Olga, "Skills of the Psychiatric Nurse," *American Journal of Nursing,* 47:174–176, 1947.

Wise, Carroll, "The Relation of the Mental Hospital to the Community," *Mental Hygiene,* 29:412–422, 1946.

Index

Acceptance, vii, 36
Alcoholics, 68-70
Alcoholics Anonymous, 70
Anxiety, 60-61
Assurance, *see* Self-assurance
Attitude
  definition of, vi, 36
  expression of, ix, x
  in nursing, vii
Attitude, nurse's
  courtesy, 97, 99
  disapproval, 26, 52, 66
  firmness, 7-8, 44-45, 56-60, 64
  friendliness
    active, 3, 4, 7, 8
    consistent, 53
    guarded, 72-73
    passive, 5, 62
  good-humored, 73
  helpfulness, 40
  in answering questions, 28-35
  in pediatric nursing, 81
  indulgence, 4
  kindliness, 59-60
  love, unsolicited, 47, 49-54, 81, 88-92
  matter-of-factness, 7, 12-14, 16, 24, 32, 43-44, 62
  naturalness, 93
  non-judgmental, 62, 72-74, 93
  non-punitive, 74-77
  patience, 66-67, 91-92
  permissiveness, 4, 41-43
  professionalism, 36
  punitive, 24-25
  sincerity of assumed, 45-47
  toward Don Juans, 73
  toward parents, 93-94
  toward psychoneurotics, 61
  toward psychotic children, 91-95
  toward schizophrenics, 50
  toward visitors, 41
  watchfulness, 6, 18-20

Birdwhistell, R. L., 104-105

Cases, 81, 84, 87, 90
  child, 79-80
  schizophrenic, 51, 58-59
Children
  as individuals, 85
  concept of time, 83
  destructiveness as curiosity, 86
  expressing anger toward, 87
  level of behavior, 82-83
  need for attention, 78
  positive approach to, 86, 92
  treasured possessions, 79-80
Children, abnormal, 78-81, 87-95
  dirtiness, 90
  hospital routines for, 87-89
  hospitals for, 81
  lack of affection, 79
  need for love, 89
  nursing-care requirements, 81
  parents, 93-94
  playrooms, 92
Cigarette lighters, 23
Conversation as a restraining technique, 27
Cosmetics, patients', 21-22

INDEX

Dangerous articles, 21-22
Dictionary of Psychology, 36
Doctor's orders, necessity for obeying, 40-42
Don Juanism, 72-73
Drug addiction, 71-72

Empathy, definition, 36

Family visits, *see* Visitors
Federal Narcotics Act, 71
Feeble-minded, 64-67
Fire prevention, 18
Firmness, 7-8, 44-45, 56-60, 64
Friendliness
  active, 3, 4, 7, 8
  consistent, 53
  guarded, 72-73
  passive, 5, 62

Guilt, feelings of, 54-56, 69, 72

Hiding places, 20
Hospital routine, 4, 63, 69, 87-89
Hospital ward organization, 15
Hospitals, psychiatric
  admission routine, 11
  personnel training, 10
  safety precautions, 18-23
  social activities, 14-15
Hydrotherapy, 24

Indulgence, 4
Infantilism in alcoholics, 69-70

Keliher, Alice, quoted, 88
Keys, 20-21
  restraint, 21
Kindliness, 59-60

Laws
  on drug addiction, 71
  on restraint, 24
Love
  as therapy, 89-90, 96-100
  as a weapon, 89
  unsolicited, 47, 49-51, 81, 88-92
Lying, 73-75

Matches, 23
Matter-of-factness, 7, 12-16, 24, 32-33, 43-44, 62
Menninger, Karl, quoted, 99
Mental illness, increase, 96

Nurse
  as group leader, 16, 99
  as hostess, 11-14, 16, 34
  as mother figure, 15-16, 25, 101
  as "paid public servant", 102, 104
  as a person, 102-103
  as "ward mama," 15-16
  as whipping boy, 75
  changing qualifications of, ix
  hostility feelings, 7
  liking for her field essential, 11, 46, 50, 61
  need for self-assurance, 28-29
  responsibilities of, 101-104
  security feelings, 6, 11
  tone of voice, 80-81
Nurse, psychiatric, necessary attitudes, 10
Nurse-patient relationships
  establishment of, 13-14
  interest in the individual, 96-99
  over-attachment, 94-95
  with Don Juans, 73

Obscene language, 33
Occupational therapist, 15
Over-attachment, 94-95

Patience, 66-67, 91-92
Patient
  acceptance of dependency, 16
  admittance to hospital, 11-14
  agitated, 57-59
  alcoholic, 68-71
  amorous, 32
  anxiety of, 60
  attempts to attract attention, 31, 33
  attitude toward hospital, 11
  child, 78-95
  childishness of, 16, 37-38
  complaining, 7, 61-62
  depressed, 7-8, 54-59
  diversionary tasks, 7-8

INDEX

Don Juans, 72-73
drug addicts, 71-72
feeble-minded, as a civic problem, 65
   teachability, 65-66
   institutionalized, 66-67
feeling of rejection, 98
frightened, 5, 8, 11-13, 29-30, 60-61
given sense of security by nurse, 37
hiding articles, 20
hostility feelings, 5, 8, 11, 38-39, 75, 98
   methods of relieving, 53-54
in a locked room, 20
lying, 73-75
need for protection, 37-39
need for self-respect, 99
personal belongings, 21-22
psychoneurotic, 61-64
questions asked by, 28-35
reaction to disapproval, 26
restraining, 8, 23-27, 38-41
schizophrenic, 8, 48-54, 75
self-punitive, 7
sensitivity, 25
special privileges for, 40-43
suicidal, 6-7, 18-23, 54-57
table manners, 26
testing reality, 29-30
thieving, 76-77
with brain damage, 67-68
Pediatric nursing, 81
Permissiveness, 4
Playrooms, 92
Psychoneurotics
   attitudes required toward, 62-64
   description, 61-64
Psychotic children, *see* Children, abnormal

Questioning by patients, 28-35
   as an aid in socialization, 34
   attention-getting, 31
   methods of answering, 31-34
   "testing reality," 30

Razors, 22
Rehabilitation of schizophrenics, 52
Rejection feelings, 98
Resocialization, 34, 52
Restraint keys, *see* Keys, restraint
Restraints
   as protection, 38
   attitudes as, 24-26
   conversation as, 29
   from outside contacts, 40-41
   laws regarding, 24-25
   mechanical, 24, 39
   sedatives for, 23
Routines, *see* Hospital routines

Schizophrenics, 8, 48-54
   day-dreaming, 49
   destructive outbursts, 53-54
   infantilism, 49
   loneliness, 48
   lying, 95
   nursing attitudes required, 49-54
   rehabilitation, 52
Sedatives as restraints, 23
Self-assurance in nurse, 28-29
Social workers, 41
Straitjackets, 24
Success, definition, vi
Suicides, 6, 18-23, 54-57
Sympathy
   definition, 36
   expression of, ix

Tactfulness, 64, 75, 76
"Testing reality" by patients, 29-30
Thieving, 76-77

Visitors, 40-41
   nurse's relationship to, 41

"Ward mama," 15
Warren, Howard C., 36
Watchfulness, 6, 18-20, 57-58, 72, 77
Work as a therapeutic agent, 56-57

INDEX

Don Juans, 72-73
drug addicts, 71-72
feeble-minded, as a civic problem, 65
  teachability, 65-66
  institutionalized, 66-67
feeling of rejection, 98
frightened, 5, 8, 11-13, 29-30, 60-61
given sense of security by nurse, 37
hiding articles, 20
hostility feelings, 5, 8, 11, 38-39, 75, 98
  methods of relieving, 53-54
in a locked room, 20
lying, 73-75
need for protection, 37-39
need for self-respect, 99
personal belongings, 21-22
psychoneurotic, 61-64
questions asked by, 28-35
reaction to disapproval, 26
restraining, 8, 23-27, 38-41
schizophrenic, 8, 48-54, 75
self-punitive, 7
sensitivity, 25
special privileges for, 40-43
suicidal, 6-7, 18-23, 54-57
table manners, 26
testing reality, 29-30
thieving, 76-77
with brain damage, 67-68
Pediatric nursing, 81
Permissiveness, 4
Playrooms, 92
Psychoneurotics
  attitudes required toward, 62-64
  description, 61-64
Psychotic children, *see* Children, abnormal

Questioning by patients, 28-35
  as an aid in socialization, 34
  attention-getting, 31
  methods of answering, 31-34
  "testing reality," 30

Razors, 22
Rehabilitation of schizophrenics, 52
Rejection feelings, 98
Resocialization, 34, 52
Restraint keys, *see* Keys, restraint
Restraints
  as protection, 38
  attitudes as, 24-26
  conversation as, 29
  from outside contacts, 40-41
  laws regarding, 24-25
  mechanical, 24, 39
  sedatives for, 23
Routines, *see* Hospital routines

Schizophrenics, 8, 48-54
  day-dreaming, 49
  destructive outbursts, 53-54
  infantilism, 49
  loneliness, 48
  lying, 95
  nursing attitudes required, 49-54
  rehabilitation, 52
Sedatives as restraints, 23
Self-assurance in nurse, 28-29
Social workers, 41
Straitjackets, 24
Success, definition, vi
Suicides, 6, 18-23, 54-57
Sympathy
  definition, 36
  expression of, ix

Tactfulness, 64, 75, 76
"Testing reality" by patients, 29-30
Thieving, 76-77

Visitors, 40-41
  nurse's relationship to, 41

"Ward mama," 15
Warren, Howard C., 36
Watchfulness, 6, 18-20, 57-58, 72, 77
Work as a therapeutic agent, 56-57